A Straight Talking Introduction to

Psychiatric Drugs

D1331560

Joanna Moncrieff

PCCS BOOKS
Ross-on-Wye

First published in 2009

PCCS BOOKS Ltd
2 Cropper Row
Alton Road
Ross-on-Wye
Herefordshire
HR9 5LA
UK
Tel +44 (0)1989 763900
www.pccs-books.co.uk

**A Straight Talking Introduction to
Psychiatric Drugs**

A CIP catalogue record for this book is available from the British Library

ISBN 978 1 906254 17 9

Cover designed in the UK by Old Dog Graphics
Typeset in the UK by The Old Dog's Missus
Printed in the UK by Ashford Colour Press, Gosport, Hampshire

Contents

Introduction to the *Straight Talking* series

What are mental health problems?

Much of what is written and spoken about emotional distress or mental health problems implies that they are illnesses. This can lead us all too easily to believe that we no longer have to think about mental health problems, because illness is best left to doctors. They are the illness experts, and psychiatrists are the doctors who specialise in mental illness. This series of books is different because we don't think that all mental health problems should be automatically regarded as illnesses.

If mental health problems aren't necessarily illnesses, it means that the burden of responsibility for distress in our lives should not be entirely shouldered by doctors and psychiatrists. All citizens have a responsibility, however small, in creating a world where everyone has a decent opportunity to live a fulfilling life. This is a contentious idea, but one which we want to advance alongside the dominant medical view.

Rather than accept that solutions to mental health problems are 'owned' by the medical profession, we will take a good look at alternatives which involve the users of psychiatric services, their carers, families, friends and other 'ordinary people' taking control of their own lives. One of the tools required in order to become active in mental health issues, whether your own or other people's, is knowledge. This series of books is a starting point for anyone who wants to know more about mental health.

How these books are written

We want these books to be understandable, so we use everyday language wherever possible. The books could have been almost completely jargon-free, but we thought that including some technical and medical terms would be helpful. Most doctors, psychiatrists and psychologists use the medical model of mental illness and manuals to help them diagnose mental health problems. The medical model and the diagnostic manuals use a particular set of terms to describe what doctors think of as 'conditions'. Although these words aren't very good at describing individual people's experiences, they are used a lot in psychiatric and psychological services, so we thought it would be helpful to define these terms as we went along and use them in a way that might help readers understand what the professionals mean. We don't expect that psychiatrists and psychologists and others working in mental health services will stop using medical terminology (although we think it might be respectful for them to drop it when talking to their patients and their families), so these books should help you get used to, and learn *their* language.

The books also contain resources for further learning. As well as lists of books, websites and organisations at the end of the book, there are endnotes. These will not be important to everyone, but they do tell the reader where information – a claim about effectiveness, an argument for or against, or a quotation – has come from so you can follow it up if you wish.

Being realistic and reassuring

Our aim is to be realistic – neither overly optimistic nor pessimistic. Things are nearly always more complicated than we would like them to be. Honest evaluations of mental health problems, of what might cause them, of what can help, and of what the likely outcome might be, are, like so much in life, somewhere in between. For the vast majority of people it would be wrong to say that they have an illness from which they will never recover. But it would be equally wrong to say that they will be completely unchanged by the distressing thoughts and feelings they are having. Life is an accumulation of experiences. There is usually no pill, or any other treatment for that matter, that will take us back to 'how we were before'. There are many things we can do (and we will be looking at lots of them in this series) in collaboration with doctors, psychiatrists, psychologists, counsellors, indeed everyone working in mental health services, with the help of our friends and family, or on our own, which stand a good chance of helping us feel better and build a constructive life with hope for the future.

Of course, we understand that the experiences dealt with in these books can sometimes be so overwhelming, confusing and terrifying that people will try to escape from them by withdrawing, going mad or even by trying to kill themselves. This happens when our usual coping strategies fail us. We accept that killing oneself is, in some circumstances, a rational act – that for the person in question it can make a lot of sense. Nonetheless, we believe that much of the distress that underpins such an extreme course of action, from which there can be no turning back, is avoidable. For this reason, all of the books in this series point towards realistic hope and recovery.

Debates

There is no single convenient answer to many of the most important questions explored in these books. No matter how badly we might wish for a simple answer, what we have is a series of debates, or arguments more like, between stakeholders and there are many stakeholders whose voices demand space in these books. We use the word 'stakeholders' here because service users, carers, friends, family, doctors, psychologists, psychiatrists, nurses and other workers, scientists in drug companies, therapists, indeed all citizens, have a stake in how our society understands and deals with problems of mental health. It is simultaneously big business and intimately personal, and many things in between. As we go along, we try to explain how someone's stake in distress (including our own, where we can see it), whether business or personal, can influence their experience and judgement.

Whilst we want to present competing (sometimes opposing) viewpoints, we don't want to leave the reader high and dry to evaluate complicated debates on their own. We will try to present reasonable conclusions which might point in certain directions for personal action. Above all, though, we believe that knowledge is power and that the better informed you are, even though the information might be conflicting, the more able you will be to make sound decisions.

It's also useful to be reminded that the professionals involved in helping distressed people are themselves caught in the same flow of conflicting information. It is their *job*, however, to interpret it in our service, so that the best solutions are available to as many people as possible. You may have noticed that the word 'best' brings with it certain challenges, not least of all, what we mean when we use this term. Perhaps the best means the most effective? However, even using words like 'effective' doesn't completely clear up the puzzle. An effective treatment could be the one which returns someone to work quickly, if you are an employer, or one which makes someone feel happier and more calm, if they are your son or daughter. Readers will also know from recent press coverage that the National Institute for Health and Clinical Excellence (NICE) which evaluates and recommends treatments, keeps one eye on the budget, so 'effective' might mean 'cost effective' to some people. This brings us to evidence.

Evidence

Throughout these books there will be material which we will present as 'evidence'. This is one of the most contentious terms to be found in this series. One person's evidence is another person's fanciful mythology and yet another person's oppressive propaganda. Nevertheless the term crops up increasingly in everyday settings, most relevantly when we hear of 'evidence-based practice'. The idea behind this term is that the treatments psychologists and psychiatrists offer should be those that work. Crudely put, there should be some evidence that, say, talking about problems, or taking a prescribed drug, actually helps people to feel better. We encounter a real problem however, when trying to evaluate this evidence, as the books will demonstrate. We will try not to discount any 'evidence' out of hand, but we will evaluate it, and we will do this with a bias towards scientific evaluation.

The types of evidence that will be covered in these books, along with their positive and negative points, include the following.

Research methods, numbers and statistics

On the one hand, the logic of most research is simple, but on the other hand, the way things have to be arranged to avoid bias in the results can lead to a perplexing system of measurements. Even the experts lose the sense of it sometimes. We'll try to explain the logic of studies, but almost certainly leave out the details. You can look these up yourself if you wish.

The books in this series look at research into a wide range of issues regarding mental health problems, including the experience of distress, what is known about the causes of problems, and their prevention and treatment. Different research methods are more or less appropriate for each of these areas, so we will be looking at different types of research as we go along. We say this now because many readers may be most familiar with studies into the *effective treatments* of distress, and we want to emphasise that there are many credible and valid sources of essential information about distress that are sometimes overlooked.

You may have come across the idea that some research methods are 'better' than others – that they constitute a 'gold standard'. In the case of research into the effectiveness of different treatments, the gold standard is usually considered to be 'randomised controlled trials' (RCTs). In simple terms, RCTs are complex (and often very expensive) experiments in which a group of individuals who all suffer from the same problem are randomly allocated to a treatment or a 'control' condition (at its simplest, no treatment at all) to see whether the treatment works. We are not necessarily convinced that RCTs always *are* the best way of conducting research into effective treatments, but they are, at the present time, the method given most credence by bodies which control funding, such as the National Health Service's National Institute of Health and Clinical Excellence (NICE), so we need to understand them.

Personal experience

Personal experience is an important source of evidence to the extent that nowadays, people who have suffered debilitating psychiatric distress are sometimes called 'experts by experience'.

Personal stories provide an essential counterbalance to the impersonal numbers and statistics often found in research projects such as RCTs. Whilst not everyone is average, by definition, most people are. Balancing the average results obtained from RCTs with some personal stories helps complete the picture and is now widely accepted to the extent that it has given birth to the new field of 'survivor research'.

Understanding contexts

Widening our view to include the families and lives of people, and the cultural, economic, social and political settings in which we live completes the picture. Mental health problems are connected to the conditions in which we all live, just as much as they are connected to our biology. From the start we want readers to know that, if there is one message or model which the books are trying to get across, it is that problems in mental health are more often than not the result of complex events in the environments in which we live and our reactions to them. These reactions can also be influenced by our biology or the way we have learned to think and feel. Hopefully these books will help disentangle the puzzle of distress and provide positive suggestions and hope for us all, whether we work in the system, currently have mental health problems ourselves, are caring for someone or are friends with someone who has.

We hope that readers of these books will feel empowered by what they learn, and thereby more able to get the best out of mental health services. It would be wonderful if our efforts, directly or indirectly, influence the development of services that effectively address the emotional, social and practical needs of people with mental health problems.

Richard Bentall
Pete Sanders
April 2009

Chapter 1
The place of drug treatments in psychiatry

Drugs of various sorts are the mainstay of modern psychiatric treatment and have been since about the 1950s. Most people who receive psychiatric services are prescribed one sort of psychiatric drug, and often several. General practitioners prescribe such drugs to many millions of other people they classify as suffering from psychiatric or psychological disorders. Indeed, the taking of psychiatric drugs dominates the whole of psychiatric services. Relations between mental health professionals and service users often revolve around medication. For example, professionals spend much time persuading people to take medication they do not want to take, tweaking doses if something goes wrong, adding drugs and changing drug regimes. Misfortunes are usually attributed to patients not taking their medication or having the dose reduced, even where there are other perfectly plausible explanations. In many cases there is no clear evidence that people are any better off since they were prescribed their array of psychiatric drugs than they were without them.

The publicity given to the benefits of psychiatric drugs like Prozac and Ritalin, and the idea that people with psychiatric problems have 'chemical imbalances', have persuaded many people that they need psychiatric drugs in order to be normal. Hence the pressure to prescribe psychiatric drugs now comes not just from professionals but also from patients, and potential patients, who have become convinced that they have a brain disorder and that drugs offer a solution to their difficulties. This has been a boon for the pharmaceutical industry, which has seen sales of antidepressants rocket since the early 1990s, and sales of 'mood stabilisers', 'antipsychotics' and stimulants starting to follow suit. Psychiatric drugs have become pharmaceutical bestsellers, making important contributions to drug company profits.

Even before the 1950s, drugs, especially sedatives, were used extensively in psychiatric hospitals and prescribed to outpatients. However, they received little attention because they were generally regarded simply as a means of chemical restraint.[1,2] It was other procedures such as ECT (electro-convulsive therapy) and insulin coma therapy as well as psychosocial interventions that were thought of as the important treatments at this time. However during the 1950s and 1960s a new range of drugs was introduced into psychiatry and views about how they worked gradually transformed. They came to be seen not simply as inducing useful but crude states of sedation and passivity, like the older style drugs, but as acting to reverse underlying psychiatric diseases.

The nature of psychiatric disorder has been contested for as long as psychiatry has existed. The psychiatric profession, being a branch of the medical profession, has continually tried to justify its dominant role by the assertion that madness and psychological distress are essentially the same as other medical problems like lung cancer and gout. But competing explanations and approaches have always existed both outside and within psychiatry. The view of psychiatric disturbance as a disease of the brain or body has constantly been challenged by some recipients of psychiatric care, but in the 1960s the antipsychiatry movement articulated philosophical and political objections to the very concept of psychiatric disorder as a medical illness.[3] How to best help sufferers has also been contested. In the early days of psychiatry, the psychosocial approach known as 'moral treatment' was well respected. Moral treatment was based on the idea that mad people could learn to control their behaviour with the right guidance. It was pioneered at an asylum run by and for Quakers called the York Retreat. Psychoanalysis, other forms of psychotherapy, social interventions and psychological approaches have also competed with or been practised alongside mainstream biological psychiatry at one time or another.

However, over the last few decades the biological view of psychiatric problems has strengthened. In the same way that the symptoms of asthma, for example, are known to be produced by tightening up of the air passages in the lung, it is assumed that the problems that are labelled as psychiatric conditions like depression and schizophrenia are caused by particular dysfunctional processes located in the brain. This view of the nature of psychiatric disorders has helped justify widespread prescription of drug treatments to people with all manner of psychiatric difficulties. In turn the assumption that drugs act by reversing an underlying disease has helped strengthen the notion that psychiatric disorders are caused by discrete biological defects.

It is sometimes apparent that the development of a market for certain drugs has shaped our views about the nature of psychiatric disorders and even brought new disorders into being. For example, the modern concept of depression was not widely accepted until the development of the idea of an antidepressant drug.[4] Prior to the introduction of drugs that were considered to be antidepressants (but which probably act in quite different and varied ways, as explained in Chapter 5), depression was regarded as a serious and rare condition, usually only encountered in people with severe manic depression or in the elderly. When the existence of antidepressant drugs was first suggested, drug companies set about popularising the view that depression is a common disorder that is not just found in psychiatric hospitals but in many other settings. They also suggested that it was frequently unrecognised. More recently, as psychiatrist David Healy has documented, the concept of depression has been expanded even further to create a large market for the SSRI (selective seratonin re-uptake inhibitors) antidepressants like Prozac.[5] Drug companies have also promoted little known conditions such as 'social anxiety disorder', 'panic disorder', 'intermittent explosive disorder' and 'compulsive buying disorder' alongside efforts to market their products. In this way the pharmaceutical industry has helped to create psychiatric diseases out of problems that were previously viewed as arising from social or interpersonal situations and may not even have been regarded as problems at all.

The pharmaceutical industry has been influential in shaping the modern landscape of psychiatric treatment in other ways as well. It conducts a majority of the research on psychiatric drugs, including most of the trials that supposedly establish whether a drug is effective and beneficial or not. As will be explained in Chapter 3, there are many ways in which the results of trials can be massaged to produce the right message. A recent study found that 90% of trials comparing different antipsychotics found a result that favoured the sponsoring company's product, leading to contradictory results.[6] For example, a study sponsored by the makers of X would generally favour X over Y but a study that was sponsored by the makers of Y would favour Y over X.

Aims

In this book I will challenge the erroneous assumption that underpins the current use of psychiatric drugs: the assumption that drugs reverse an underlying medical disease. I will then present an alternative approach to the use of psychiatric drugs that emphasises the fact that they are psychoactive substances that induce states of intoxication. I believe this view provides a better way of assessing the balance between possible benefits and harmful effects of drugs. After describing the different theoretical approaches to understanding how psychiatric drugs work, I will look at the evidence for the effects of the main classes of psychiatric drugs that are currently used, including the neuroleptics or 'antipsychotic' drugs; 'antidepressants'; 'mood stabilisers' or drugs used for manic depression; stimulants; and benzodiazepines. Throughout the book I have had to make use of terms that I do not necessarily endorse. The names of some drugs reflect a presumption that they act in a disease-specific way, but this whole book challenges that presumption. However, terms that make this presumption have become commonly used as in the case of 'antipsychotic' and sometimes, as with the term 'antidepressant', there is no readily available alternative. Hence I have had to use these terms occasionally, although I have avoided them where possible. Similarly, the idea that psychiatric disturbance is a medical illness is so entrenched in our culture that it is difficult to avoid the use of medicalising language, such as illness, treatment and patient. Alternatives are often clumsy and their meaning is not always clear. Therefore I have retained the use of this language in much of this book for the sake of simplicity and readability, but this should not be taken as an acceptance of its full medical implications.

Chapter 2
How do psychiatric drugs work?

Do drugs treat psychiatric diseases?

As described in the previous chapter, Western psychiatry
portrays the behavioural disturbances and emotional suffering
that it deals with as diseases. It suggests that these disturbances
arise, like other diseases, from a disruption in the smooth
running of some part of the body, usually the brain. Over the
last two centuries there have been numerous attempts to
identify the physical causes of madness and distress, with
different theories going in and out of fashion. The idea that
psychiatric disorders are genetically transmitted has been
popular for a long time and over the last few decades birth
complications, viral illnesses, structural brain defects and
imbalances in brain chemicals have all been proposed to be the
cause of mental disorders.

Because psychiatric problems are believed to be diseases, it is
usually assumed that the major types of drug used in psychiatry
work by reversing or partially reversing the underlying disease
process. We find that the naming of psychiatric drugs reflects
this assumption; so 'antipsychotics' are thought to act on the
biological abnormality that produces symptoms of psychosis or
schizophrenia, 'antidepressants' are thought to reverse the basis
of depressive symptoms, 'mood stabilisers' are thought to help
rectify the process that gives rise to abnormal fluctuations of
mood and 'anxiolytics' are thought to address the biological
mechanism that creates anxiety. Stimulants are said by many to

specifically counteract the basis of hyperactivity or 'attention deficit hyperactivity disorder' (ADHD), as it is now known. This view of the nature of psychiatric drugs can be called the *disease-centred model* of drug action. Although this is now the dominant view of what psychiatric drugs do, this model is actually relatively new. It developed during the 1950s and 1960s when most of the drugs we are familiar with in psychiatry were first introduced.[1]

The disease-centred model is based on the same logic that is used to explain the action of drugs in the rest of medicine. Although few medical drugs reverse the ultimate cause of a disease, most act to reverse or partially reverse part of the biological process that produces the symptoms of disease. Psychiatrists often compare the need for psychiatric drugs to the use of insulin in diabetes for example. Insulin treatment does not reverse the ultimate cause of diabetes, the failure of the pancreas gland, but it does help reverse the consequences of the disease by replacing the body's insulin supply. Other medical drugs including symptomatic treatments like painkillers act in this way. Painkillers for example counteract part of the biological processes that gives rise to pain. In this sense most drugs used in general medicine act according to a disease-centred model. This is no accident, since medical drugs are developed to target identified disease processes. Disease-centred drugs are more powerful because they target the biological mechanism responsible for the particular symptoms.

The disease-centred model of drug action is closely related to theories that state that psychiatric conditions are caused by abnormalities in particular brain chemicals, or a 'chemical imbalance'. We now know that the brain contains many chemical substances that help to transmit messages between the nerve cells that make up the brain (Figure 1).

Figure 1: *Picture of nervous transmission*

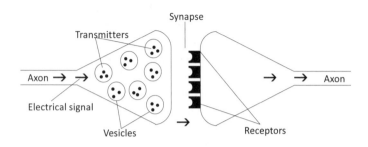

These chemicals are called 'neurotransmitters' and include substances like dopamine, noradrenalin, serotonin, acetylcholine, endorphins and many more. They are involved in helping the electrical impulse that travels along the nerves to cross the gaps between nerve cells that are known as 'synapses'. What happens is that when the electrical impulse arrives at the terminal of one nerve or neuron, it causes release of a neurotransmitter from the sacks or 'vesicles' in which it is stored. The transmitter travels across the synapse and attaches to receptors on the surface of the next neuron. The bonding between the neurotransmitter and the receptor activates (or sometimes inhibits) the nervous impulse in the second nerve cell. Some psychiatric drugs act on the receptors for a number of the neurotransmitters, either blocking or enhancing the receptors' ability to transmit impulses. The neuroleptic or antipsychotic drugs, for example, block dopamine receptors and stop the chemical dopamine from transmitting its messages in a normal fashion. Opiate drugs like heroin and morphine stimulate receptors that are usually activated by the body's natural pain-killing chemicals, the endorphins. Drugs can also affect neurotransmitters by directly stimulating their release, acting on the processes by which they are made, or acting on the mechanisms by which they are inactivated or removed from the synapse. One of the ways in which neurotransmitters are inactivated is by their re-absorption or re-uptake into the nerve cells. Antidepressants are thought to act by stopping the re-uptake and deactivation of the neurotransmitters serotonin and noradrenalin, leading to an increase in the levels of these chemicals in the synapses. However, as explained in Chapter 5 it has not been demonstrated that these drugs do reliably increase levels of these transmitters. Stimulants like amphetamine and Ritalin directly stimulate the release of noradrenalin and dopamine into the synapse and reduce their re-uptake from the synapse.

Following the observation that psychiatric drugs act on neurotransmitters systems, it began to be proposed that an abnormality in these systems might be the cause of psychiatric disorders. The best-known example of this way of thinking is the dopamine hypothesis of schizophrenia. The idea that depression is caused by a deficiency of serotonin or noradrenalin is another example, sometimes referred to as the 'monoamine theory' of depression (serotonin and noradrenalin are both classified as monoamine-type neurotransmitters). Although scientists acknowledge that these are merely theories, which are far from being proven, there is a widespread public perception that the biochemical origins of various psychiatric disorders have been clearly identified.

Is there any evidence that psychiatric disorders are caused by a chemical imbalance?

No psychiatric disorder has been conclusively linked to a single biochemical disturbance. The dopamine theory of schizophrenia and the monoamine theory of depression have been the most thoroughly researched. As far as depression is concerned, studies of serotonin and noradrenalin function show a confusing and conflicting picture, with some suggesting a deficiency, some suggesting an excess and some showing no relation.[2] Expert psychiatrists and researchers admit that no one has yet demonstrated that there is an abnormality of serotonin in depression.[3]

In schizophrenia and psychosis it is dopamine that has been the main focus of interest, although other chemicals have also been proposed to have an effect from time to time. The dopamine hypothesis of schizophrenia suggests that schizophrenia or psychosis is due to hyperactivity of the dopamine system. In its more sophisticated versions it suggests that the 'positive' symptoms of schizophrenia, or the symptoms of acute psychosis like delusions and hallucinations, are produced by overactivity of dopamine, even if the dopamine system is not the ultimate cause of the disorder. There is a little indirect and still rather inconsistent evidence of raised dopamine activity in people with acute psychosis. However, this evidence comes from comparing brain activity in people who are experiencing an acute episode of psychosis with a group of 'healthy controls'. The healthy controls are often staff or relatives of staff who work in the hospital. But the symptoms of psychosis are not the only difference between these two groups. People who are having a psychotic episode are likely to be more aroused than the controls and it may be the level of arousal that accounts for the excess dopamine activity, since we know that dopamine is associated with arousal. Studies also show that dopamine is released when an animal or human is experiencing stress, when they move about, when they pay particular attention to something, when they smoke and in response to numerous other situations. It is likely that many of these factors will differ between people with psychosis and healthy controls. People with psychosis are more likely to be agitated, anxious, stressed, hyperactive and they probably have higher rates of smoking. So many things may account for the indications of raised dopamine activity in people with psychosis that do not point to there being a specific link between dopamine and psychosis. In addition, a lot of other research has generally not shown a relationship between dopamine and psychosis or schizophrenia. For example, post-mortem examinations, the only way to measure dopamine content of the brain directly, found no difference between people with schizophrenia and controls. Some studies of dopamine receptors revealed that they were increased in the brains of people with schizophrenia, but this increase turned out to be due to the fact that the patients in these studies had been taking neuroleptic drugs on a long-term basis. These drugs block dopamine activity and it has been shown in animal studies that the brain responds to this situation by making extra dopamine receptors.[4]

Therefore even the most well-accepted biochemical theories about the origins of psychiatric symptoms and disorders have little factual support. It is often said that the effects of drug treatment is the best evidence that there is a biochemical origin to psychiatric conditions. It is argued that because drugs have biochemical effects and because they appear to benefit people with psychiatric symptoms, then the disorders must have been produced by a biochemical state that is opposite to that produced by the drugs. However, this argument can only be used if it is assumed that drugs act according to a disease-centred model, by reversing the underlying disease mechanism (or part of it). In the next section we will see that there is an alternative explanation for the action of psychiatric drugs, that I have called the drug-centred model. If this alternative model is accepted, then the effects of drugs no longer support theories that mental disorders arise because of specific disturbances in the brain's biochemistry.

An alternative model of drug action: The drug-centred model

Another way of explaining the effects of psychiatric drugs is what I have called the *drug-centred model* of drug action. Table 1 illustrates the main contrasting features of the two models.

Table 1: *Alternative models of drug action*

Disease-centred model	Drug-centred model
Drugs correct an abnormal brain state	Drugs create an abnormal brain state
The beneficial effects of drugs are derived from their effects on a presumed disease process	The drugs alter the expression of psychiatric problems through the super-imposition of drug-induced effects
Example: insulin for diabetes	Example: alcohol for social anxiety

The disease-centred model assumes that drugs exert their therapeutic effects by reversing an underlying biological abnormality or disease. In contrast, the drug-centred model says that the drugs influence the expression or symptoms of psychiatric problems by inducing an abnormal biological state. Psychiatric drugs are *psychoactive drugs*. This means they are drugs that affect the nervous system and alter the way we think and feel. The psychoactive drugs we are used to hearing about in these terms are used for recreational purposes, like alcohol and illegal drugs such as cannabis, cocaine and heroin. All these drugs make people feel and behave differently from normal when they take them. They produce what is called a state of 'intoxication' and each different type of drug produces a particular sort of intoxication, depending on what chemical effects it has on the nervous system. When these drugs are taken in large quantities the alterations they induce will be extreme and obvious. But even small doses produce a subtle impact on behaviour and experience. Psychiatric drugs are no different. They also produce characteristic states of intoxication that are different from the normal undrugged state. However, in contrast to recreational drugs, which generally make people feel good, at least in the short term, most psychiatric drugs produce states that vary from mildly unpleasant to completely unbearable.

Therefore whereas the disease-centred model assumes that psychiatric drugs help to restore normal brain functioning, the drug-centred model suggests that the drugs themselves *create* an abnormal brain state. According to the drug-centred model it is the drug-induced state that impacts on someone experiencing mental distress and it is this impact that is described as a 'response' to treatment according to the conventional disease-centred view. However, the drug-centred model suggests that taking psychiatric drugs merely substitutes a drug-induced state for the original state of mental disturbance. If the disturbance is very severe, then the abnormal drug-induced state may be regarded as preferable by the sufferer, or the people who are trying to help them.

In psychiatry, an accepted example of a drug-centred treatment is the recognised benefits of alcohol in social phobia. Alcohol can help people with social anxiety because a state of mild intoxication, feeling merry in other words, is associated with a lessening of social inhibitions. No one suggests that alcohol works by reversing an underlying biochemical imbalance or correcting an insufficiency of alcohol in the brain. Alcohol works because it substitutes the alcohol-induced brain state, with its characteristic weakening of inhibitions, for the normal anxious state.

The drug-centred model stresses that taking a drug creates an *abnormal* biological state. A drug is a foreign substance as far as the body is concerned, and the body automatically tries to get rid of it. If the body can't get rid of the drug, because the person continues to take it, the body tries to counteract its effects. This places the body under a biological stress because it is constantly straining to oppose the effects of the drug. Therefore taking a drug does not return a system that is functioning abnormally towards normal, as the disease-centred model assumes; it actually drives the body into an abnormal and biologically stressed state. In this way the drug-centred model helps to explain the harmful effects that taking any sort of drug on a long-term basis inevitably involves.

Evidence for the disease-centred model of drug action

Prior to the 1950s drugs were regarded as acting in a drug-centred way. When the neuroleptics like chlorpromazine (brand names, Largactil, Thorazine) were introduced in the 1950s, they were first regarded as having a drug-centred action. It was even suggested that they induced a neurological disease, and that they had to do this in order to be useful. The symptoms of the disease supplanted the symptoms of the psychiatric disorder.[5] However, gradually the drugs came to be seen as disease-specific treatments, and the idea that they were drugs that produced profound and unusual psychoactive states was swiftly forgotten.[6]

Psychiatry adopted the disease-centred model of drug action because it bolstered the idea that psychiatric disorders were the same as other medical conditions, and could be managed and treated in the same sort of way. The model was never tested. It was never compared to the alternative drug-centred explanation of how drugs work. The disease-centred model simply came to be assumed to be the case. People stopped considering that there could be an alternative.

For this reason, there is little evidence that would allow you to decide which model of drug action is superior. Since no one can deny that psychiatric drugs have psychoactive effects, the onus is on the proponents of the disease-centred model to justify that psychiatric drugs work through exerting a specific effect on an underlying disease process, over and above the psychoactive effects they induce. But because most researchers have simply ignored the possibility that drugs work through inducing an abnormal state of intoxication, there is little evidence which could refute the drug-centred model and establish that drugs do indeed exert a specific action on a disease process. Most research that has been conducted with psychiatric drugs since the 1950s is consistent with a drug-centred explanation of their effects in people with psychiatric conditions.[7]

An example of the lack of evidence to support the disease-centred view of drug action is the fact that there is little evidence that drugs that are meant to have specific effects in certain conditions, like antidepressants in depression, are really better than other sorts of drugs. In the rest of this book I describe some of this research in more detail, and other publications also provide more information.[8,9] Briefly, in studies of people with depression, numerous drugs (and other types of treatment) not conventionally regarded as antidepressants have been shown to have similar effects to antidepressants. Several studies of people with psychosis or schizophrenia show that other drugs like the benzodiazepines (diazepam [Valium] for example) or opium have similar effects to so-called 'antipsychotic' drugs. These other drugs have sedative actions, but they work in a completely different way on the brain from drugs conventionally regarded as antipsychotics. In particular, they do not block dopamine receptors.

Readers will have to decide for themselves whether the drug-centred or the disease-centred way of thinking about psychiatric drugs best explains their effects. In my view the drug-centred model provides the best framework for understanding what psychiatric drugs do to someone who takes them, why they might sometimes be helpful, and what harmful effects they might also produce. This model suggests that the therapeutic benefits that some psychiatric drugs appear to have are a coincidental by-product of the characteristics of the altered, drug-induced state they produce. Sometimes these effects will be worthwhile. Often however, by distorting normal bodily function, drugs have an adverse impact. They may therefore do more harm than good, particularly in the long term.

Consequences of long-term drug use

Drugs are foreign substances from the point of view of the body and therefore the body tries to counteract their effects. This is why drug addicts need to keep taking higher and higher doses of drugs like opiates or benzodiazepines to get the same buzz. This phenomenon is called 'pharmacological tolerance'. The body does this in various ways. In response to a drug that affects the activity of the brain's chemical messengers, the neurotransmitters, the body may adjust the number of receptors for that chemical or it may increase or reduce the sensitivity of the receptors. These changes can be viewed as the body's adaptations to the presence of a drug. Animal studies show that this process may begin within days of starting a drug if it is taken repeatedly on a daily basis. The consequences of this process are that the acute effects of drugs diminish and larger and larger doses are required to obtain the same effects. If the drug is stopped then the body's adaptations are suddenly unopposed by the presence of the drug, and they give rise to withdrawal symptoms, which will persist until the body has returned to normal and the adaptations have disappeared. However, readers may be surprised to learn that we have little knowledge about the body's response to psychiatric drugs. The full range of bodily adaptations that different psychiatric drugs induce has not been adequately studied. We also have little information about how long it takes for the body to recover its normal structure and function after a drug is stopped and whether the drug-induced changes are reversible or not.

The trouble is that the changes or adaptations that the body makes to try and counteract the effects of drugs are unpredictable. They do not necessarily simply balance out the effects of the drugs. For example, the disorder called tardive dyskinesia consists of involuntary movements and possibly other neurological impairments (see Chapter 4). It is known to be caused by prolonged use of drugs that block dopamine activity such as the neuroleptic or antipsychotic drugs. The symptoms are thought to result from overactivity of the dopamine system as the body tries to oppose the effects of these drugs. Dopamine activity is associated with increased movement and especially with involuntary or compulsive movements like those seen in tardive dyskinesia. Therefore in tardive dyskinesia the body's adaptations do not simply balance out the dopamine-blocking effects of the drugs, but overdo it. This results in too much dopamine activity creating the abnormal movements that are characteristic of the condition. The mechanism of tardive dyskinesia is probably more complex than this, and has not been worked out completely, but the principle that drug-induced adaptations can be maladaptive and dysfunctional is important.

Long-term use of drugs may also cause effects that directly damage brain cells. Several recent studies suggest that the long-term use of neuroleptic drugs is accompanied by a reduction in brain cell matter and a corresponding increase in the volume of the brain cavities or ventricles. These studies will be described in more detail in Chapter 4. Again there is little research on how long-term exposure to psychiatric drugs might directly affect the nerve cells of the brain and the mechanisms of any effects are not known.

Chapter 3
Interpreting the evidence on psychiatric drugs

In subsequent chapters I will summarise some of the large amount of research into the effects of different classes of psychiatric drugs. This research is difficult to interpret for a number of reasons. First, psychiatric drug research uses the methods that are applied to the study of treatments for physical diseases. However, as mentioned earlier, many people have challenged the validity of treating psychiatric problems as if they were medical or bodily conditions. Viewing a psychiatric problem as a medical disease or disorder suggests that it can be identified, quantified and measured independently of the person who is experiencing the problem. This is the way that we talk about the characteristics of cancer of the liver or heart disease or arthritis. We can measure the features of these conditions fairly easily because they are physical and because they have similar characteristics in all the different people who have them. But measuring non-physical things like emotional experiences, thought processes and behaviours is more complex. This is because it is more difficult for people to agree on what they think about them. For example, how do we decide whether person X is more sad than person Y? One observer may feel that X's behaviours and statements indicate greater sadness, but another may believe that it is Y who shows the deepest emotional distress. In addition, it is difficult to understand emotional states, thoughts and behaviours as abstract entities. They always 'belong' to someone, to an individual person, and it is difficult to see what they really mean if they are considered independently from the people who experience them. Sadness, for example, is not a thing that can be weighed and measured in its own right. There is always a person who is sad, and to understand sadness, we need to understand the situation of the individual who is suffering.

What this all means is that measuring the symptoms of mental disorders as if they were the symptoms of physical diseases is not necessarily helpful. It does not tell us anything about the real nature of a person's problems. Emotional states and behaviours cannot be described and quantified in the same way that we measure the properties of physical objects. Therefore when measuring scales and scores are used to describe mental states in psychiatric research it is not clear what they really mean, or indeed if they mean anything at all.

Second, as mentioned in the previous chapter, most research involving psychiatric drugs is conducted on the assumption that the disease-centred model of drug action is correct. Since this model was adopted in the 1960s it has barely been questioned and is so well accepted that most psychiatrists are not even aware that there are other ways of considering the effects of psychiatric drugs. Therefore most research on psychiatric drugs does not attempt to describe the sort of state of intoxication that they produce, and the consequences of such a state. Instead, research studies simply assume that drugs reverse an underlying disease process and attempt to measure the 'symptoms' of the 'disease'. Therefore any changes that are observed are assumed to be changes in the disease. In this situation the obvious mental alterations produced by most psychoactive drugs are ignored and interpreted as changes in the underlying disorder.

Third, research is highly influenced by groups whose interests are best served by overstating the benefits of drugs. The psychiatric profession and the pharmaceutical industry conduct and publish most research on drug treatments. Both these institutions have reasons to underplay the adverse effects of drugs, overstate their benefits and promote a disease-centred model of drug action. An example of how these groups can influence research is what is known as 'publication bias'. This refers to the fact that studies that find positive effects of drugs are more likely to be published than studies that find that drugs have no benefits or cause harm. Researchers in Sweden, for example, showed that studies of antidepressants were more likely to be published if they showed a superior effect of antidepressants over placebo and studies that found no difference were sometimes not published at all.[1] In addition, most studies look at several different measures of benefit or outcome. Published reports of studies often emphasise the measures that show the drug in the best light.[2] Measures that show no benefit or that indicate harmful effects may not be published or may be concealed in the small print of the article. Some pharmaceutical companies have been shown to withhold data that does not show their drug in a favourable light.[3] But doctors, researchers and editors have also played a part in focusing on research that highlights the positive and plays down the negative effects of drugs.

These problems suggest that most of the research concerning the effects of psychiatric drugs on psychiatric patients is meaningless. It uses instruments that measure intangible personal experiences as if they were material objects, and it ignores the fact that psychiatric drugs are psychoactive substances that alter normal brain function in ways that are bound to interact with psychiatric problems. In addition, the biases of the people who conduct and write up research may easily distort how research is presented. Although they are so highly regarded, randomised controlled trials in psychiatry are problematic since they import a design that was devised to assess the impact of treatments on physical conditions without consideration for the issues involved in assessing human behaviours and experiences. They also ignore the impact of drug-induced effects. However, despite these problems expert committees that produce guidelines, like the National Institute for Health and Clinical Excellence (NICE) in the United Kingdom, are influenced by existing research evidence and particularly by the results of randomised controlled trials. The way that psychiatrists prescribe medication is also increasingly determined both by guidelines and by their understanding of the research evidence. Therefore it is important to understand the principles of how research on psychiatric drug treatments is conducted in order to understand its results. This also puts people in a better position to judge the value of advice that is issued about psychiatric drugs.

Randomised controlled trials (RCTs)

Figure 2: *Randomised controlled trial design*

Start by defining people who might receive the treatment to be tested (for example people with depression for a trial of a treatment for depression) – **the population**

Select a **sample** for the study (often younger and older people are excluded, as well as people with other conditions, like physical illness)

Randomly divide the sample into groups

Give groups the **different treatments** to be studied (e.g. in a placebo-controlled trial, one group is given the drug and the other the placebo)

Measure and compare the **outcomes** of the different groups

Before randomised trials became the mainstay of drug evaluation, many treatments were assessed by starting the treatment and seeing how people progressed. If they improved it was often said that the treatment had worked. This interpretation might be appropriate if you were certain that the condition was going to deteriorate, but many conditions in psychiatry and medicine have a fluctuating course. In fact most psychiatric disorders improve spontaneously, at least from time to time. Therefore it is necessary to separate the effects of the treatment from the way the condition might normally progress. It was for this reason that 'controlled' trials were devised. In controlled trials people are divided into groups: one group is given the treatment that is being researched and one group, the control group, is not. Both groups are then followed up for a period of time and their outcome is compared.

Randomised controlled trials are controlled trials where participants are allocated to the different groups at random. Usually this is done by using random number tables or computer-generated random numbers. Randomisation is recommended in order to ensure that there are no important differences between the groups. This is done because otherwise researchers might select people with a better outlook (that is, people who would get better anyway) to have the experimental treatment and consign all the people with a poor outlook to have the control treatment. Or it could be the other way round. The point is that if the groups have been chosen selectively, any differences in outcome cannot simply be attributed to the effects of the treatment. So randomisation is applied in order to ensure that, before the treatment is started, participants who have the treatment and those that are in the control group do not differ in any important way that might affect their subsequent progress.

In addition to the safeguard of randomisation, most RCTs attempt to create a situation in which people in the different groups have a similar experience throughout the course of the trial. Ideally, the only difference between the control group and the treatment group will be the actual treatment that is being tested. Therefore the control group should be given the same general aspects of treatment as the group who receive the specific treatment, such as spending time with professionals and researchers, having blood tests and filling in questionnaires. In drug trials people in the control group are also usually given a 'placebo'. This is a dummy tablet that is made of something like chalk that has no active effects. The placebo is given to mimic what are called the 'placebo' or 'non-specific' effects of taking a drug. These are the positive expectations that many people feel when they are given drug treatment. We know that, in some conditions, these expectations can themselves make people feel better. For example, some people in severe pain report that their pain improves after being given an injection of saline or water, if they are told that the injection is really of a pain-killing drug.[4]

Professionals might also be influenced by their expectations of the benefits of a new drug, and so the use of a placebo helps to prevent the staff who treat the patient, and the researchers who assess the patient, from knowing who is getting the drug treatment and who is not. Otherwise researchers may be influenced by their expectations of the value of drug treatment when they make their ratings of outcome. They might be inclined to rate someone they know is taking the drug as doing better than someone who is not, for example, even when there is no real difference between them. When a placebo is used in this way a trial is described as being 'double blind'. This means that the patients and the researchers are blind to the nature of the treatment they receive. In other words no one knows, or is supposed to know, who is getting the real drug or who is getting the placebo tablet.

Because double-blind randomised controlled trials are carefully designed to minimise the influence of things like selection and the effects of expectation, they are often referred to as the 'gold standard' of treatment research. Large trials especially are regarded as providing reliable evidence on the benefits or otherwise of treatments and guideline committees give them a lot of weight. Meta-analyses are also regarded as providing high-quality evidence. A meta-analysis is a combination of the results of a number of different trials of the same treatment. But in fact meta-analyses are as good or as poor as the trials that they combine, a fact that is sometimes overlooked. By combining studies meta-analysis is a powerful instrument that can yield results that look strongly positive. But a meta-analysis of poorly conducted trials, as well as adding together their results, also summates their deficiencies or biases. The result of a meta-analysis may therefore be more misleading than the original studies.

Randomised controlled trials are designed to indicate whether the drug being tested improves the outcome of the condition being treated more than the 'control' treatment. In a trial comparing a drug with a placebo, the groups are compared on a measure of outcome, such as the score on a depression rating scale. Statistical tests are applied to see if there is a genuine difference between the scores of the two groups. If the difference is big enough, and the study has enough participants, then the probability that the difference just occurred by chance will be low. When the probability, or the p value as it is also known, is less than 5%, or 0.05, then we say by convention, or agreement, that the result is statistically significant. This means that we accept that there is a real difference between the outcome of the two groups. However, although conventionally the result is accepted as real, 5% of the time it will still occur by chance. If for example, we do 100 tests, or use 100 different measures of outcome (as many studies do), then even if there is no real difference between the groups, on average five of our results will be 'statistically significant'.

Problems with randomised controlled trials of psychiatric drugs

1. *Influence of drug-induced effects*

Because of the assumption that drugs act in a disease-centred fashion, randomised controlled trials have not attempted to control for the *pharmacological* effects that drugs induce. Taking a psychoactive drug produces effects such as sedation and a feeling of being drugged or slow. These effects may change people's experience and behaviour without affecting the underlying problem. For example, many antidepressants have sedative effects. These effects will help people sleep, they may reduce anxiety and they may simply make someone feel so groggy that they no longer feel depressed. All these factors may be interpreted as an improvement in depression, but none implies that there is any real change in the individual's underlying emotional state.

2. *Unblinding*

The use of a placebo tablet is meant to prevent people from knowing whether they are getting the real drug or not. It is based on the assumption that people cannot distinguish between an active drug and a totally inert tablet. However, it is often quite easy for people in trials to tell whether they are taking the drug or the placebo. If the drug has any psychoactive properties, then it will make people feel different in some way. People will notice effects such as sedation and grogginess, for example, or they may notice physical effects such as a dry mouth or nausea. People on placebo might be anticipating some drug-induced effects, and notice that they do not experience any. The chance that people will detect whether they are taking a drug or a placebo is heightened because people who take part in trials are given detailed information about the process of the trial and the nature of the drug being tested, including its side effects. Thus people are well aware that they might get a drug or they might get a placebo, and are often keen to try and decide which they have been allocated. They are also well aware of what sort of effects the real drug might produce.

What this suggests is that many trials that are supposed to be double blind are probably not double blind at all. Many of the participants and some of the professionals involved are likely to be able to work out who is taking the real drug and who is on the placebo. In fact trials in which people are asked to guess what they are taking show that in most cases people can detect the nature of the pill they have been given.[5] If people taking part in trials believe that drugs are likely to help them, which they often do or they would not have agreed to take part, they may have a heightened expectation that they will improve if they suspect they are taking the real drug. Similarly they may have lowered expectations if they believe they have been given the placebo. Hence the levels of expectations that people have about their treatment will differ between the drug and the placebo or control group. In this case any differences in the outcome of treatment may be due to these different expectations rather than the effects of the drug.

3. *Medication withdrawal effects*

Since modern psychiatric drugs were introduced in the 1950s they have been prescribed on a long-term basis for many patients. Therefore, when investigators first wanted to look at whether long-term drug treatment was really beneficial, they found that most of the subjects they wanted to recruit were already taking long-term treatment. However, it did not occur to them that this might be a problem, and they simply randomised half of the subjects to have their drugs replaced by a placebo tablet. Therefore, trials of long-term treatment in most cases do not compare people who have been newly started on a drug with people who try to manage without drug treatment. They involve people who are already taking long-term drug treatment and they compare people who are continued on this treatment with people who are suddenly withdrawn from it.

The problem with this design is that we know that withdrawing from any sort of psychoactive drug has a number of adverse effects.[6] These are described in more detail in Chapter 10, but briefly they include:

1. physical withdrawal symptoms
2. withdrawal-related psychosis
3. withdrawal-induced relapse
4. psychological effects

What this means is that people who are placed on placebo in trials of long-term drug treatment are liable to suffer from one or more of these withdrawal-related effects. Therefore if they appear to deteriorate, and their outcome is not as good as people who continue to take their medication without interruption, this does not establish that the medication has helped prevent a relapse of their underlying disorder. It may simply be that they are experiencing withdrawal symptoms. Since these commonly include insomnia and agitation, they may easily be mistaken for relapse. Alternatively people may develop a psychotic withdrawal reaction to some types of drug including neuroleptics, or they may suffer a relapse of their psychiatric condition that is precipitated by the stress of withdrawal. There is good evidence for all these situations, which is covered in more detail in Chapter 10. People may also become psychologically dependent on taking medication and feel anxious and vulnerable if they believe it has been stopped. The point I am making here is that studies that compare people who have just had their medication discontinued with people who continue to take it cannot demonstrate that taking medication in the first place helps to improve outcome. It only shows that after someone stops medication there may be a number of difficulties, which may give the appearance that they have deteriorated. In many cases the deterioration will not be a full relapse of the previous psychiatric condition, but merely the predictable physical and psychological consequences of drug withdrawal.

4. Analysis and presentation of trials

There are numerous ways in which the results of trials can be massaged to inflate the effectiveness of drugs and to play down their adverse effects. As discussed earlier, measures that give positive results can be published and ones that show negative results suppressed. For example, one old study of depression used almost 700 measures.[7] As explained above (p. 24), on average one in twenty results will be positive just by chance, using statistical tests, without there being any real beneficial effect. The published reports of this study presented the few positive measures without acknowledging the number of measures that had been made and the likely explanation that the positive results were simply chance findings.

The way data is analysed can also affect results. Grouping people into either 'responders' or 'non-responders' may give the impression that there is a large difference between the people who have taken the drug and people who have taken the placebo, for example. However, this may conceal the fact that the actual difference between the groups, in terms of the rating scale scores used to do the grouping, was very small.[8]

5. Dropouts from trials

Many people who enrol in drug trials subsequently drop out. That is they stop taking their allocated treatment, they stop attending assessments, or they relapse and require additional treatment. At this point their involvement in the trial is usually terminated. The problem with this is that we do not know the ultimate outcome for this group of people. For example, an individual may drop out at a time of crisis, and appear to be doing badly on their allocated treatment, but then subsequently improve. In a case like this, the data obtained for the purposes of the trial will not provide a good assessment of how this person has fared over the full course of the trial period. In addition, if people allocated to the active drug treatment drop out for different reasons than people taking placebo, this may unbalance the outcomes of the groups and invalidate the results of the trial.

Drug-centred evaluation of drugs

These problems, and particularly the fact that research has overlooked the profound psychoactive effects that psychiatric drugs produce in all people has led researcher David Cohen to claim that conventional randomised controlled trials are completely useless.[9] They do not even begin to tell us what sort of effects psychiatric drugs produce. In other words if we accept a drug-centred account of how psychiatric drugs work, evidence from randomised controlled trials cannot help us much. What we need are different sorts of studies. First of all we need studies with volunteers, that is people without psychiatric problems, to allow researchers to characterise the global effects that a drug induces. In these studies we need descriptions of how the drug affects people from the volunteers themselves, and also from friends and family who know the person well. We need to know what it feels like to take the drug, how the drug affects arousal, mental processes and emotional reactions. We also need information about what the drugs does to bodily functions like heart rate, blood pressure and levels of various hormones. We need this information over long periods, since we know that the effects that drugs have after they have been taken for some time may be different from the effects they exert if they are just taken once or twice. It is also important that the people who take the drug have an opportunity to comment on what it felt like to take it after they have stopped taking it. Sometimes people think they are functioning well on a drug, and only realise when they look back how impaired they actually were.

However, few such studies exist. Therefore, at present, information about what effects drugs induce has to be gleaned from anecdotal reports and from looking at data on what are designated as 'side effects'. According to a disease-centred model, side effects are any effects other than the effect on the disease process itself. According to a drug-centred model, drugs effects cannot be parcelled off in this way and effects that are currently written off as side effects may give us important clues as to what sort of global state a drug induces. Only when we know the characteristics of this state, can we start to figure out how it might impact on various sorts of psychiatric problems.

In the following chapters I will describe what is known about the global effects that different psychiatric drugs induce. I will then provide an overview of existing research on the benefits of the drugs, bearing in mind that it was mostly conducted from a disease-centred point of view. I will also consider evidence of major adverse effects. I will then discuss what benefits might be obtained from the use of the different sorts of drugs and what considerations might be involved in deciding whether or not to use them.

Chapter 4
Neuroleptic drugs (also known as 'antipsychotics' and major tranquillisers)

The term 'neuroleptic' refers to a group of drugs that are associated particularly with the treatment of psychosis and schizophrenia. They are also known as 'antipsychotics', but I have avoided the use of this term where I can because it implies that they have a specific action, that they can reverse the causes of psychosis. This chapter will suggest that they work in a different, drug-centred way.

The term 'neuroleptic' comes from the Greek and means to seize hold of the nervous system. As will become clear below, this is a useful description of the action of these drugs. As well as being used for psychosis and schizophrenia, neuroleptic drugs are also used in a range of other situations, particularly to calm and subdue people who are agitated or aggressive. Therefore they are also prescribed to people who are diagnosed with mania, personality disorder, dementia, learning difficulties, autism, anxiety, depression and other disorders. The first drugs of this sort were introduced in the 1950s and 1960s and are now sometimes referred to as 'first generation', 'typical' or just older neuroleptics. Beginning in the 1990s a new range of these drugs has been introduced which are known as 'atypical' or 'second generation' neuroleptics or antipsychotics.

How do they work?

The conventional view is that the drugs reverse the chemical imbalance that is suggested to be the cause of the symptoms of schizophrenia or psychosis. Most neuroleptic drugs strongly counteract the effects of the brain chemical called dopamine. As explained earlier (p. 9), this led to the hypothesis that psychotic symptoms are produced by overactivity of dopamine. Hence the disease-centred view of the action of neuroleptics suggests that they work by correcting, or partially correcting, an underlying abnormality in the dopamine system.

In contrast, a drug-centred view of the action of these drugs suggests that they do indeed produce a characteristic state of dopamine deficiency and that this state can be useful in some psychiatric situations. However, this is not because the drugs correct an underlying overactivity of dopamine. As described in Chapter 1 (pp. 10–11), studies that have compared levels of dopamine and its receptors in people with psychosis and schizophrenia with levels in healthy people have found little evidence that there is a specific abnormality of dopamine activity in these conditions. A drug-centred model suggests that a state of dopamine deficiency such as that produced by these drugs can suppress the symptoms of psychosis, as well as reducing levels of physical disturbance and high arousal *by suppressing all mental and physical activity.*

So what sort of state do the neuroleptic drugs produce? The global neurological effects of these drugs were clearly described by the psychiatrists who first used them back in the 1950s. They induce a neurological state that is similar to Parkinson's disease. Parkinson's disease is a disease caused by degeneration of the cells in the area of the brain that produces dopamine (the substantia nigra) and its symptoms reflect a reduction of the activity of the dopamine system. Dopamine has a stimulatory effect on a part of the brain called the basal ganglia, a group of cell bodies buried deep in the brain matter in the stem of the brain. The main characteristics of reduced dopamine activity are a reduction in movement and a general slowing up of mental processes.

Neuroleptic drugs have similar effects. They cause people to move less and their movements become slower. Reduced movement in the facial muscles causes people to show less facial response and they develop a typically blank facial expression. Emotional responses are also reduced. Emotional experiences like sadness and happiness are less intense and people who have taken these drugs describe feeling emotionally flattened, indifferent or numb. The drugs slow up people's thinking and make it especially difficult for people to make themselves do things. This is referred to as having difficulty with 'initiating actions' and even simple things like responding to questions may become difficult. Some tasks that would usually be straightforward may seem just too much effort. Two Israeli doctors who took an injection of haloperidol for experimental purposes described how they were unable to read, use the telephone or perform household tasks of their own will, but could do so if instructed to by somebody else.[1] Getting sandwiches from a sandwich machine was too daunting for a volunteer in another study who took a dose of an old neuroleptic drug called droperidol.[2] Most of these drugs also have sedative activity and make people sleepy. Peter Breggin, an American psychiatrist and well-known critic of psychiatric drugs, summarises the effects of these drugs as a state of 'deactivation', a term which captures the restriction of physical and mental activity that they produce.[3]

Numerous studies which have measured the mental abilities of volunteers who have taken neuroleptic drugs show that the drugs slow up or impair people's mental functioning in some way. When people have taken a dose of these drugs they have difficulty with co-ordination, attention, learning and memory, and they have slower reaction times and slower movements.[4,5] Studies with laboratory animals also find that animals that are given these drugs have difficulty performing their usual activities and show impaired learning and memory.[6]

Like Parkinson's disease the neuroleptic drugs cause obvious physical signs such as making people's muscles very stiff, especially at higher doses. Drugs are less likely to cause the tremor that is typical of Parkinson's disease however. At lower doses the characteristic muscle stiffness may be absent or only very subtle. Therefore people are often only diagnosed as having what are referred to as Parkinsonian side effects, or extra-pyramidal side effects when they are on relatively high doses of neuroleptic drugs.

Figure 3: *Extra-pyramidal system*

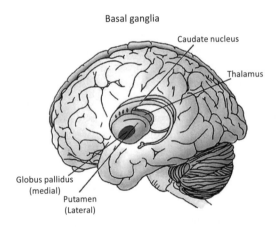

Basal ganglia

Caudate nucleus

Thalamus

Globus pallidus
(medial)

Putamen
(Lateral)

The extra-pyramidal system is named to distinguish it from the pyramidal-shaped bundles of fibres that carry messages about voluntary movement between the body and the brain. The extra-pyramidal system consists of fibrous tracts that lie below the main body of the brain. These fibres are influenced by input from various areas of the brain including the substantia nigra and the basal ganglia. The extra-pyramidal system is involved in reflexes, locomotion, complex movements, and postural control. There are links between the extra-pyramidal system and areas of the brain that control thinking, initiative and emotions. Important transmitters in the extra-pyramidal system include dopamine, acetylcholine, GABA and glutamate.

However, lower doses do produce less obvious signs of Parkinson's disease, like slower movements and loss of the normal range of facial expression. It is logical that the blockade of dopamine will cause a continuum of symptoms. We know from animal studies that at very high doses dopamine-blocking drugs produce a state in which animals are rigid and unable to move, although still conscious. This state is referred to as 'catalepsy'. At moderate to high doses they cause the typical signs of Parkinson's disease, that is muscular rigidity, physical and mental slowing and flattened emotions. At lower doses there is no reason to believe that these processes are not present in a milder form.

As well as the deactivation effects, most neuroleptics appear to induce a state of intense restlessness. This state is called *akathisia* and it is usually an extremely unpleasant experience. People feel compelled to move about and have a feeling of psychic tension or anxiety. This effect is commonly referred to as an extra-pyramidal effect because it is thought to be produced by effects of the drugs on the basal ganglia or extra-pyramidal system. However, the exact mechanism by which it occurs remains unclear.

So how could this drug-induced state be useful in dealing with psychiatric or psychological problems? A drug-centred account of the action of antipsychotic drugs suggests that it is the Parkinson's disease-like state that they produce that is responsible for their apparently useful effects in psychosis and other psychiatric disorders. In this sense they act as a chemical straightjacket that has both physical and mental actions. They reduce physical movement and arousal, which may be useful in people who are hyperactive or aggressive. They usually make people sleep more than usual, which may be helpful in someone with severe insomnia. Their 'antipsychotic' effect is achieved by their ability to suppress all mental activity. Since they slow up all mental processes they help to suppress abnormal thoughts and experiences such as delusions and hallucinations. Therefore they may be useful for the symptoms of acute psychosis or what are known as the 'positive symptoms' of schizophrenia. However, there is no evidence that they are selective for abnormal thoughts, and accounts by people who have taken these drugs for a variety of problems indicate how they affect all mental processes.[7]

It is not clear from a drug-centred account how the effects of neuroleptics could be helpful for what are called 'negative' symptoms of schizophrenia.

Figure 4: *Positive and negative symptoms of schizophrenia*

Positive symptoms	Negative symptoms
Hallucinations	Reduced speech
Delusions	Reduced motivation
Feelings of being controlled	Social withdrawal
Feelings of having thoughts read, broad-cast or interfered with	Blunted emotions
Incoherent or tangential speech	

Most psychiatrists acknowledge this. Indeed, the effects of neuroleptics are similar to the negative symptoms of schizophrenia. Negative symptoms include apathy, reduced motivation and emotional flattening. All these features can also be a consequence of taking neuroleptic drugs and studies show that they can improve when neuroleptic drugs are reduced.[8] However, some people with 'positive' symptoms or acute psychotic symptoms may exhibit negative symptoms because they are so preoccupied with their internal mental experiences that they withdraw from social interaction and become physically inactive. In such people the drugs may be able to enhance their physical and social activity by suppressing their mental processes. However, it is difficult to see how the more long-term defects in motivation observed in some people with a diagnosis of schizophrenia could be helped by 'deactivating' drugs.

Effects of discontinuation

Neuroleptics are sedative drugs that decrease the activity of the nervous system. The nervous system tries to counteract their effects by, for example, producing more dopamine receptors. When the drugs are withdrawn the brain's adaptations make the nervous system overactive until the body has re-adapted to not having the drug present anymore. Thus people who withdraw from neuroleptics have reduced sleep and become physically agitated. They are also likely to become mentally aroused or anxious. Other physical effects of the drugs may be seen in reverse. The drugs reduce gut motility, causing constipation (similar drugs are used to combat nausea and sickness). Therefore withdrawal is often associated with nausea and diarrhoea and occasionally with vomiting. As explained further in Chapters 3 and 10, withdrawal can occasionally induce psychotic symptoms.

Old versus new antipsychotics

Some of the newer antipsychotic drugs are thought to work in the same basic way as the old ones, by blocking dopamine activity and producing a state of mild Parkinson's disease. Risperidone, for example, causes overt Parkinson's symptoms at moderate to high doses. However, others may act differently, although we are not yet sure how. Olanzapine and clozapine appear to induce Parkinson's-type symptoms only at much higher doses and yet at lower doses they still have a strong sedative effect that is associated with the suppression of psychotic experiences like delusions and hallucinations. People taking clozapine in particular often spend much of their time asleep, they are often calmer and in some cases less obviously troubled by their inner thoughts. Another very characteristic effect of both drugs is that they stimulate appetite and cause people to put on substantial amounts of weight. In fact they appear to have a general disruptive effect on the body's metabolic systems. Both these drugs affect a wide range of brain chemicals, including noradrenalin, histamine, serotonin and acetylcholine as well as dopamine. We are not sure how they produce their effects, but their impact on any or all of these chemical systems may contribute.

Evidence for their usefulness

Short-term use in psychosis and schizophrenia

Several placebo-controlled randomised trials show that neuroleptics reduce the general disturbance in people who have an acute psychotic episode. They also reduce the strength of abnormal experiences like delusions and hallucinations to a greater extent than placebo. This should come as no surprise given what we know of their general effects. However, whether they are superior in these respects to other sorts of sedative drugs is less certain. For example, an old randomised controlled trial that compared an old neuroleptic called chlorpromazine (Largactil or Thorazine) to opium in people with acute psychosis showed that people improved to the same extent with both drugs over the three weeks of the study.[9] Seven studies have compared benzodiazepine drugs like diazepam (Valium) and lorazepam to various neuroleptics.[10] Three of these studies found that the neuroleptic was superior, three that the benzodiazepine was superior and one was inconclusive. The main effect of benzodiazepine drugs is sedation, so it may be the reduction of arousal and activity that accounts for their benefits. However, several studies demonstrated that, like neuroleptics, they reduced psychotic symptoms like delusions and hallucinations as well. In contrast two studies that compared early neuroleptics with barbiturates, another type of sedative drug, found that the neuroleptics were superior.[11,12]

So the studies show that, on average, in the short term neuroleptic drugs reduce the impact of psychotic symptoms and other manifestations of acute psychotic episodes better than a placebo. However, it is not clear whether they are superior to other sedative drugs.

The next question is whether everyone who is given these drugs benefits to the same extent and whether there might be people who do just as well without the drugs. In the 1970s there was some interest in these questions, but more recently they have been neglected. In the 1970s Loren Mosher, an American psychiatrist, set up the Soteria project in San Diego, California. This was a small homely unit designed to care for people with psychotic disturbance or schizophrenia, avoiding the use of neuroleptic drugs if possible. The outcome of people who entered the Soteria project was compared to the outcome of a similar group of people who were treated in conventional psychiatric hospitals. Results showed that people who entered the Soteria project did as well as the comparison group and that they used far fewer drugs. 30% of people randomised to Soteria avoided the use of neuroleptic drugs altogether.[13] A more recent study in Finland of people with a first psychotic episode also found that 43% of people could be successfully managed without using any neuroleptic drugs.[14] So a third or more of patients with an episode of psychosis may recover without the need for neuroleptic drugs.

It is also widely recognised that another 30% of patients remain disturbed despite the use of these drugs. People in this situation are sometimes said to have 'treatment-resistant' schizophrenia and it is these people for whom clozapine is recommended. Studies that compare clozapine with other neuroleptics (mainly haloperidol) for people in this situation have found that clozapine is superior at least in the short term, although longer studies show a lesser effect.[15] Clozapine is reserved for treatment of people in whom other treatments have failed because of the risk of developing a life-threatening blood disorder called agranulocytosis. This is a condition in which the white blood cells are drastically reduced, which compromises the body's immunity and can cause death by inhibiting the body's ability to fight infection.

Clozapine may help a proportion of people who fail to respond to other drugs, but we know that sadly many of these people continue to experience some symptoms and difficulties. Therefore, it may be that only a minority of people who experience an acute psychotic breakdown get benefit from taking neuroleptic drugs. We also don't know whether neuroleptics are superior to other types of sedative drugs in this situation.

Long-term use for relapse prevention

Neuroleptics are taken on a long-term basis both by people who have fully recovered from a psychotic episode and by people who experience continuing symptoms to some degree. In the first case, long-term drug treatment is recommended because it is believed to reduce the chances that someone will suffer a relapse. In the second situation drug treatment is continued because it is believed that the person would be worse off without it. Ongoing drug treatment is believed to be necessary to reduce the intensity of the symptoms. Many studies have not distinguished these situations very clearly, and most involve people from both categories.

As explained in Chapter 3 (pp. 26–9), randomised controlled trials of long-term treatment for people diagnosed with psychosis and schizophrenia involve selecting people who have already been taking neuroleptic drugs, usually on a long-term basis, and switching half of them onto a dummy tablet or placebo. These people are highly likely to experience withdrawal symptoms and they are vulnerable to all the other adverse effects associated with withdrawal of neuroleptic medication including withdrawal-related psychosis (supersensitivity psychosis) and withdrawal-induced relapse. Therefore the mental state and behaviour of many of the people in the placebo group is likely to deteriorate as a consequence of drug withdrawal, quite apart from any effect due to the underlying condition. But this has been almost completely unrecognised in studies of long-term treatment. Any deterioration is therefore simply labelled as a relapse.

What this means is that existing research studies are not able to tell us whether taking neuroleptic drugs on a long-term basis is better than not taking them from the point of remaining mentally well. All they indicate is that people who are withdrawn from long-term medication, especially if the withdrawal is rapid, experience more problems overall than people who continue to take it – which is not the same thing.

I must point out that there is an overwhelming consensus that people who have psychotic episodes or schizophrenia should take medication on a long-term basis to prevent relapse or deterioration. In practice most patients are recommended to stay on these drugs for the whole of their lives. However, it is my belief that the use of long-term drug treatment is not supported by reliable evidence. This is because the research studies have ignored the adverse consequences of withdrawing from previous medication in people who are placed on placebo. This is not the same as saying that drug treatment is definitely unhelpful. But we simply do not have the evidence on which to make a reliable judgement about its efficacy in this situation. There are no studies that can tell us whether taking neuroleptic drugs on a long-term basis is superior to not taking them in the first place or taking them briefly with a slow and careful withdrawal. In addition, existing studies tell us mainly about relapse rates and most have ignored other aspects of outcome, like people's overall ability to function, their ability to work, to have relationships and to enjoy their lives.

Many people will have had the experience of seeing someone who has been taking these drugs relapse or deteriorate soon after stopping them. It seems as if this proves the necessity of taking the drug and certainly this convinces most mental health professionals of the need for long-term drug treatment. What I have been pointing out is that a relapse or deterioration after stopping neuroleptic drugs may be a consequence of the process of withdrawal from the drug, rather than the re-emergence of a prior disorder. Long-term drug treatment may be beneficial, but if it is we do not know the size or extent of its benefits. Alternatively, it may have no prophylactic value at all. It may simply be the case that long-term psychiatric medication is difficult to stop. Evidence suggests that if withdrawal is done slowly and carefully, the risk of developing problems after withdrawal is lower.[16]

Long-term use for symptom suppression

The other potential justification for long-term drug treatment is with people who have ongoing continuous psychotic symptoms. Although most people recover at least somewhat from an acute psychotic episode, some remain severely disturbed, and some of those who improve continue to experience some residual symptoms and difficulties. Since neuroleptic drugs can suppress psychotic symptoms in some people in the short term, using them on a continuing basis may be of benefit to people who experience these difficulties on a protracted basis. However, as explained in preceding chapters, we know that the body attempts to counteract the effects of foreign substances. Unfortunately, this phenomenon has not been seriously considered or much studied in relation to drugs used in psychiatric treatment. Hence there is little research that could help to show whether it occurs and to what extent. However, we do know that the use of neuroleptic drugs causes a compensatory increase in the number and sensitivity of the particular type of dopamine receptor that they block (the D_2 receptor).[*] A recent animal experiment showed that the characteristic effects of neuroleptics on animal behaviour reduced over time.[17] Therefore, it is likely that drug-induced mental deactivation also reduces with prolonged use. Increasing the dose may temporarily restore the effects of the drug, but in time the body will counteract the higher dose also.

In addition, studies which may be cited to support the efficacy of long-term treatment in preventing deterioration in people with chronic symptoms are the same studies that are quoted for relapse prevention. These studies involve people who have ongoing symptoms as well as people who have completely recovered from an acute episode of psychosis. The same considerations about the adverse effects of discontinuation of previous drug treatment in the placebo group apply in the situation of symptom suppression in someone with chronic symptoms. Discontinuing previous treatment in people who are placed on placebo may produce a deterioration due to withdrawal symptoms, including occasional psychotic withdrawal symptoms (supersensitivity psychosis), discontinuation-induced relapse and other adverse effects. Therefore people who are put on placebo may appear to get worse, and this has usually been interpreted as a worsening of their original condition. However, it may simply be the consequences of having their previous medication withdrawn.

Therefore it is difficult to know whether neuroleptic drugs are useful when taken on a continuous basis in people who have ongoing symptoms such as delusions and hallucinations. Any ability they might have to suppress these symptoms initially

---

[*] Several types of dopamine receptor have been identified. So far at least four types are known.

may well be lessened as the body adapts to their use. Studies that are supposed to support their use in this manner are flawed because the effects of drug discontinuation in people taking placebo have been ignored.

Some psychiatric researchers have suggested that prolonged use of these drugs may worsen symptoms of psychosis. The proposed explanation for this is that net dopamine activity levels may actually be increased by the body's response to the presence of a dopamine-blocking drug. This is also believed to be the explanation for tardive dyskinesia, the movement disorder produced by long-term neuroleptic use. This situation, sometimes called 'tardive psychosis', has also been called 'supersensitivity psychosis', after the suggestion that it is brought about by increased sensitivity of the dopamine receptors. However, its existence has not been proven and while so few people are treated without these drugs, it will remain difficult to demonstrate whether deterioration in some people with schizophrenia is caused by long-term drug use or is part of the process of schizophrenia itself.

Use of neuroleptics in other situations

The physical effects of neuroleptics make them useful to control aggressive and troublesome behaviour. Therefore they are prescribed to older people with dementia who sometimes become agitated and to people with learning disabilities. They are prescribed to people with anxiety, partly for their sedative effects. Their ability to slow down and suppress thought may also be useful for people with anxiety. They are sometimes prescribed to people with depression, often to help with accompanying anxiety. They are also sometimes prescribed to people diagnosed with personality disorder. There has been a worrying increase in levels of prescribing of these drug to children and young people over recent years.[18] In the majority of cases the children were not psychotic, suggesting the drugs may be employed as a general measure of behavioural control.[19] There is little evidence that the use of neuroleptic drugs produces any ultimate benefits in any of these situations.

Common adverse effects

• *Extra-pyramidal 'side effects':* This is the term used to describe symptoms produced by the effects of the drugs on the extra-pyramidal system of the brain. These include the *Parkinson's disease-type* symptoms of muscle stiffness, slowness of movement and thought. Sometimes a sudden and severe *dystonic reaction* can occur. This is when the muscles become rigid and can occur rapidly after taking the drug. It most often affects the head and neck muscles and it is frightening, painful and can occasionally be dangerous since it may paralyse the muscles of the throat leading to choking and, infrequently, the breathing muscles. Around 10% of people treated with older neuroleptics develop a dystonic reaction. It is most common in young men. Fortunately it is easily treated by giving a dose of an anticholinergic drug such as biperiden or procyclidine, which counteracts the dopamine-blocking effects of the neuroleptics. It is rarely fatal, although infrequently it can be. Akathisia is also categorised as an extra-pyramidal side effect, although the exact mechanism whereby it is produced is unknown. It is difficult to treat, and has not been shown reliably to respond to any additional drug treatment.

• *Neuroleptic malignant syndrome:* This is an uncommon reaction that occurs in around 0.5% of people newly started on neuroleptics. It is probably caused at least in part by effects on the extra-pyramidal system, but again the exact mechanism is not known. It consists a sudden reaction in which people have a high temperature and muscular rigidity. The risk of death is estimated to be around 20% and there is no specific treatment.

• *Tardive dyskinesia:* This is a syndrome that occurs after long-term use of neuroleptics. Its hallmark is the presence of involuntary movements, such as lip smacking, tongue movements or facial twitches. It usually affects the face but can involve other muscle groups. It can be permanent. This means it may sometimes persist after the drugs are stopped. It is also probably due to the effects of the neuroleptics on the extra-pyramidal system. It is thought to occur because of overcompensation of the dopamine system, possibly by increased number and sensitivity of dopamine receptors, although it is likely to involve other factors as well. As well as the abnormal movements, several studies suggest that mental deterioration is part and parcel of the syndrome of tardive dyskinesia.[20] This has led some experts to conclude that tardive dyskinesia is a condition of drug-induced brain damage that is manifested in abnormal movements *and* in a decline in mental abilities like that found in dementia.[21] Other neurological diseases involving abnormal movements like Huntingdon's chorea and Parkinson's disease also involve mental impairment, so this should not be surprising. Mainstream psychiatric literature mostly ignores this aspect of tardive dyskinesia and there has been little attempt to research it further. It is generally estimated that at least 20% of patients on older neuroleptics develop tardive dyskinesia if they take the drugs on a long-term basis.[22] It occurs more frequently in the elderly. It may be less common with use of the newer neuroleptic drugs, but this has yet to be determined conclusively.

• *Structural brain changes:* Two recent studies suggest that the use of neuroleptic drugs for weeks or months is associated with a reduction in the quantity of nerve cells in the brain, known as the 'grey matter'.[23,24]

• *Effects on the heart:* All neuroleptic drugs can cause a defect in the ability of the heart muscle to conduct electrical impulses.

This can be detected through abnormalities on the electrocardiogram (ECG), a trace of the heart's electrical output. In particular the drugs can cause prolongation of part of the heart's cycle of activity (the QT interval) and they can cause irregular heartbeats or arrythmias. These effects can lead to sudden death in people taking neuroleptics.

• *Metabolic abnormalities:* All neuroleptics can cause people to gain weight, which can predispose people to develop diabetes and coronary heart disease. Olanzapine and clozapine cause substantial weight gain in most people who take them. They also cause a noticeable increase in appetite and craving for sweet foods. This appears to be part of a general effect that involves a disruption of the body's normal metabolic processes and may be caused by drug-induced resistance to insulin, the hormone that regulates the body's metabolism. Consequences include increased risk of diabetes and raised cholesterol.

• *Hormonal abnormalities:* Dopamine inhibits the production of the hormone prolactin. Therefore reducing dopamine activity leads to an increase in prolactin levels. This is the hormone that stimulates production of breast milk, and high levels can result in breast growth in men, lactation, infertility, impotence, reduced sex drive, and the bone-wasting condition, osteoporosis. Prolactin should be measured regularly to make sure it is within safe limits. Some drugs like clozapine and quetiapine are said not to raise prolactin.

• *Other adverse effects:* Many neuroleptics counteract the activity of the transmitter acetylcholine and produce what are called 'anticholinergic effects'. These include symptoms such as dry mouth, blurred vision and constipation. Many of the drugs cause postural hypotension, which consists of a dangerous drop in blood pressure on standing and is due to the effects of these drugs on a type of noradrenalin receptor. Many neuroleptics can cause epileptic fits, and clozapine is the worst in this regard. Clozapine can also cause a dangerous drop in the white blood cells that provide the body's immunity from infection, causing conditions known as neutropaenia and agranulocytosis. Agranulocytosis is especially dangerous and can rapidly lead to death from common infections. Everyone who takes clozapine requires regular monitoring of their blood cells to ensure that this effect is detected rapidly and that clozapine is stopped immediately if it is.

• *Increased mortality:* Several studies have shown that people who use neuroleptic drugs on a long-term basis are more likely to die than the general population. Although some of this increased risk of dying is likely to be due to the lifestyle of long-term psychiatric patients such as high rates of smoking and lack of exercise, some studies indicate that the drugs play a role, even after taking account of these lifestyle factors. Being on more than one sort of neuroleptic drug is associated with a particularly high risk of early death.[25]

What is wrong with the way neuroleptics are currently used?

Despite their formidable adverse effects, neuroleptic drugs are prescribed widely and their use is increasing. In my opinion, they are being prescribed to too many people, for too long, often at overly high doses. A recent review showed that most drugs are routinely being used at doses that are way above those that have been shown to be most clinically effective.[26] A government survey conducted in 2007 estimated that one in three psychiatric patients was taking higher doses of psychiatric drugs than they needed.[27] Currently neuroleptics are given to most people who start to experience psychotic symptoms. It is very rare that someone who experiences psychotic symptoms is helped to recover on their own. This is despite the fact that we know from historical studies and from modern projects that have deliberately minimised the use of drugs, that at least a third of people can recover without neuroleptics. Only a decade ago it was accepted practice to withhold neuroleptic treatment from someone with a first episode of psychosis in order to make a clear diagnosis and in some cases to allow time for symptoms to resolve without medication. This practice has become less common and there is an increasingly widely held assumption that drug treatment is always a good thing.

There is for example an ever-burgeoning literature on the benefits of early intervention for psychosis, and on the ethically dubious practice of using antipsychotic drugs to prevent the onset of psychosis in young people. A perception is developing that early drug treatment can prevent the most serious consequences of schizophrenia. But this perception is based on a flawed interpretation of a well-known observation. It has been known for a long time that people whose psychosis develops in a slow and gradual fashion have a more severe and debilitating condition and are less likely to make a full recovery than people whose symptoms come on suddenly. This well-known fact has been repackaged and it is now suggested that it is the 'duration of untreated psychosis', in other words the delay in getting treatment, that determines the outcome of schizophrenia or psychosis. But people whose psychosis develops gradually will tend to come forward for treatment later in the course of their psychosis. Therefore, a long 'duration of untreated psychosis' can simply indicate that there has been a slow onset, a fact that is known to predict a generally poorer outcome. There is no evidence to justify the transformation of concern with the type of onset to the delay in treatment. The psychiatric community has stopped talking about the link between onset and outcome, and started talking about how to ensure that people start treatment earlier. This is just one example of an increasing inclination over the last few years to play up the benefits of drug treatment and overlook its downside.

Another assumption is that acute episodes are easily treatable and should only last a few weeks at most. If symptoms have not at least faded within this time, there is pressure to increase the dose of the neuroleptic being used, add another one or start clozapine. Part of this pressure comes from the shortage of acute hospital beds. It is also a result of the general impatience of professionals and a need to actively intervene rather than to wait for, and foster, a natural recovery. But psychotic episodes may last a long time and still resolve on their own. People who would have made a recovery in their own time are being put onto high-dose drug regimes and started on clozapine, because the mental health system is no longer prepared to wait for a natural recovery to occur.

So people are being started on neuroleptic drugs who may not need them, and this includes an increasing number of children. A good proportion of people who become psychotic may recover without the use of neuroleptic drugs, given the right help and support. People who might benefit from the temporary use of these drugs are being given overly high doses and, as stated earlier, millions of people around the world are being persuaded to take neuroleptic drugs for years on end on the basis of evidence that is fundamentally flawed.

Weighing up when to use neuroleptics

Neuroleptics, or antipsychotics, are powerful drugs. Most of them produce a state that is similar to Parkinson's disease in which people's physical actions and mental processes are slowed up and restricted. These effects may be useful in suppressing abnormal mental experiences like delusions and hallucinations and in controlling disruptive behaviour.

For each individual, the decision about whether to take neuroleptic drugs, or whether to stop taking them once they are started, depends on a fine balance between many considerations. For someone who is tortured by hallucinations and locked in their own world of mental preoccupations, they may have startling and useful effects. Many users of these drugs testify that the drugs helped suppress the abnormal mental world they were absorbed in and helped them to rejoin reality. However, this benefit comes at a high price. Most people find the experience of taking these drugs unpleasant. They do not like having their thoughts slowed up, their body slowed down and their emotional life flattened out. Akathisia is also a very unpleasant state and other 'extra-pyramidal side effects' such as muscular rigidity are disliked. The drugs that have the least propensity to cause these effects, olanzapine and clozapine, appear to work by disrupting the body's metabolism, causing phenomenal weight gain in some cases and diabetes and other abnormalities that are likely to increase the risk of heart disease in the long term. Elevation of prolactin has disagreeable effects and all neuroleptics are potentially dangerous for the heart. They have been shown to be associated with reduced lifespan. As if this were not enough, use of neuroleptic drugs has been shown to reduce brain volume to a noticeable extent on brain scans after only a few months. After several years of use they may cause a neurological disorder known as tardive dyskinesia, which involves abnormal involuntary movements probably accompanied by mental impairment. Worst of all, this condition may be permanent, that is, it may persist after the drugs are withdrawn.

Long-term use of these drugs is not justified by the evidence. Although theoretically ongoing drug treatment might be useful in people who experience persistent symptoms, we are not certain whether the useful effects of neuroleptics are maintained, or whether the body adapts to counteract them. It is also often difficult to tell whether an individual is really better after they start taking a certain drug than they were before. Even if there were evidence that long-term neuroleptic treatment was beneficial, the consequences are so severe and debilitating that it may be preferable to suffer more frequent relapses or higher levels of symptoms than to have to endure the drug treatment.

People who refuse to take long-term medication are usually labelled as difficult and non-compliant, but they may be making a perfectly rational decision based on their negative experience of drug therapy. However, coming off long-term medication can be a difficult process, as described in Chapter 10. Rather than being dismissed as being difficult, people who want to stop medication should be given support to minimise the complications of doing so. One of the problems with coming off psychiatric drugs is that there are deeply held assumptions that the drugs are indispensable. A more optimistic and supportive attitude might enable more people to withdraw from their drug treatment successfully.

Chapter 5
'Antidepressants'

During the 1950s certain drugs were tried out on people who were depressed and they began to be called 'antidepressants'. One group of drugs that were similar in structure to some of the early neuroleptics was called the tricyclic antidepressants. Another group of drugs was known as the monoamine oxidase inhibitors or MAOIs. These were the main types of antidepressant used until the late 1980s. Prozac was launched in 1988 and was the first of a series of new antidepressants introduced onto the market during the 1990s called the 'selective serotonin re-uptake inhibitors' (SSRIs). These were joined by other sorts of drugs also branded as antidepressants (including venlafaxine, mirtazapine and moclobomide).

Since their introduction, antidepressants have been prescribed by psychiatrists and general practitioners to people they diagnose as having 'depression'. From the beginning of the 1990s strenuous advertising campaigns and professional publicity increased the prescribing of these drugs substantially. Prescriptions issued increased by 234% between 1992 and 2002 in Great Britain, for example.[1] In 2002 11% of American women and 5% of men were taking an antidepressant drug.[2] Whereas once there was a great stigma attached to taking psychiatric medicines, nowadays taking antidepressants is considered to be quite ordinary and mundane.

What effects do antidepressants produce?

Based on a disease-centred approach, the conventional view of antidepressants suggests that they help correct a chemical imbalance that is presumed to be present in depression. They are said to increase the availability of particular neurotransmitters that are thought to be deficient in those suffering from depression. Older drugs, like the tricyclic antidepressants and the MAOIs were thought to act by increasing the availability of the neurotransmitter noradrenalin. The SSRIs are thought to improve depression by correcting a deficiency of serotonin. Therefore, most research on the biochemical actions of antidepressant drugs has focused on their effects on the serotonin and noradrenalin systems. However, most of these drugs affect numerous other neurotransmitters as well. Animal research on how antidepressants affect noradrenalin and serotonin levels is confusing and inconsistent. For example, some research suggests that tricyclic antidepressants reduce rather than increase noradrenalin activity.[3,4,5,6] Similarly, there is no consistent data on how SSRIs impact on serotonin transmission after long-term use.

There has been little effort to characterise the overall psychoactive effect of antidepressants and as a consequence we are hardly even aware of the features of intoxication associated with these drugs. However, a few points need to be made. Antidepressants come from many different chemical classes and therefore can be expected to vary in the effects they produce. Some tricyclic antidepressants, for example, appear to be similar in their nature to the more sedative type of neuroleptics such as chlorpromazine (Largactil), especially amitriptyline and clomipramine. Since they are usually used at doses far lower than doses of neuroleptics, dopamine-blocking effects may be less obvious, but some animal studies suggest that they have the ability to block dopamine activity in the same way as neuroleptics.[7] The predominant effect that people notice when they first take these drugs is sedation. They increase sleep and cause drowsiness during the day. They do not make people 'high'. Studies with healthy volunteers show that taking tricyclic antidepressants makes people slower in their reactions, and impairs intellectual abilities such as attention and memory. Taking them is usually an unpleasant experience for volunteers.[8,9]

SSRIs appear to have few noticeable effects in volunteer studies apart from their effects on the gut. This is not surprising, given that most of the body's serotonin is present in the gut and only a small proportion is in the brain. SSRIs commonly cause nausea and sometimes diarrhoea and vomiting. They also commonly produce mild drowsiness, but in contrast to the tricyclics they can cause insomnia rather than increased sleep in volunteers. Volunteers either report that they feel no different after taking an SSRI or they find the effects unpleasant, especially when they are given higher doses.[10]

Anecdotal reports suggest that SSRIs may have an emotional blunting effect but this has not been adequately investigated. It is impossible to say, for example, whether there is a characteristic state of emotional blunting induced by SSRIs, as there appears to be with neuroleptics. By creating a drug-induced state of altered consciousness, all psychoactive drugs, including alcohol and nicotine, are likely to make people less sensitive to the world around them. Therefore all psychoactive drugs can be said to distort our emotional experience to some extent. No research has attempted to investigate whether SSRIs have a particular type of effect on emotional experience that distinguishes them from other psychoactive substances. In fact no research has addressed this issue with any psychiatric medication. The effects of neuroleptics on emotional responses are only known from early descriptions of their effects and the testimonies of people who have tried them.

In research trials conducted with patients, a proportion of the subjects who take SSRIs develop an unpleasant state of agitation and restlessness.[11] Because of this reaction, and their ability to cause insomnia, they are sometimes said to have 'activating effects'. These activating effects appear to be similar to the akathisia induced by neuroleptics and it has been suggested that it is these unpleasant activating effects that may induce people to take suicidal or even homicidal actions.[12] However, it should be stressed that their profile of effects is not like the classical stimulant drugs such as amphetamines, which markedly increase arousal, heart rate and blood pressure and are associated with feelings of euphoria.

There are numerous other sorts of antidepressants with a variety of chemical structures and pharmacological actions. Trazadone and mianserin are older and strongly sedating drugs. Venlafaxine is a newer drug similar to the SSRIs but claimed to have noradrenalin uptake-blocking activity as well. Moclobamide is an MAOI-type drug that is claimed to avoid the dangerous interactions associated with the older MAOIs. Some antidepressants have genuine stimulant actions, that is, they increase arousal. One of the older MAOIs, tranylcypromine, had a stimulant profile, as does possibly the more recently launched drug reboxetine.[13]

Effects of discontinuation

It is now well recognised that long-term use of antidepressants results in physical and psychic symptoms when the drugs are discontinued. The nature of the symptoms varies according to the properties of the different sorts of drug. The intensity of the withdrawal syndrome depends in part on how quickly the drug is dispelled from the body. Drugs that are eliminated rapidly cause more severe withdrawal symptoms, as the body has no time to re-adjust to their absence.

Withdrawal of tricyclic antidepressants causes nausea, chills, muscle pain, insomnia and excess dreaming. MAOI withdrawal is characterised by irritability, agitation, movement disorders, insomnia *or* excessive sleep, and vivid dreams. SSRI withdrawal typically involves 'shock-like' sensations, dizziness, insomnia, irritability, excessive dreaming and weepiness. Paroxetine and venlafaxine are reputed to cause the most intense and distressing withdrawal symptoms among the SSRI and SSRI-like drugs because of their short duration of action and rapid elimination time.

Evidence for their usefulness

Short-term use

There are hundreds, maybe thousands of trials that have compared various antidepressants with placebo in people who have been diagnosed with depression. Overall most of the studies report that, by the end of the study, people taking the antidepressant have lower levels of depression than people taking the placebo. However, many studies find no difference between people on the antidepressant and people on the placebo pill. In addition, recent trials show that the size of the difference between antidepressants and placebo is very small. It is so small in fact that it is unlikely to be worthwhile even if it has a real antidepressant effect. For example, in an analysis which combined the results of several American trials of SSRIs and other new drugs, the difference between the drugs and the placebo was less than two points on the Hamilton Rating Scale for Depression.[14] This is a commonly used scale that usually has 17 items and scores up to 54 points. A difference of two points is not considered to be clinically worthwhile and may easily be produced by sedative effects (see below). Another analysis of recent trials conducted by the National Institute of Health and Clinical Excellence (NICE) found that the difference in depression scores between people randomised to antidepressants and people randomised to placebo was so small that it was, in the words of the Institute's report 'unlikely to be of clinical significance'.[15]

From a drug-centred perspective, there are many explanations of why there might be a small difference between antidepressant drugs and placebo that do not imply that the drugs specifically reverse depression. First, depression often involves insomnia or sleeping difficulties and sometimes involves anxiety and agitation. Any drug with sedative properties will improve this aspect of the problem. The Hamilton Rating Scale for Depression contains three items on sleep alone and these items can score up to six points. So any difference between drugs and placebo may reflect the sedative qualities of many commonly used antidepressants.

Second, any drug that alters our consciousness or that creates a state of intoxication may obscure or suppress depressive feelings. In other words it is difficult to feel depressed if you are feeling heavily drugged. In addition, drugs like the neuroleptics flatten out emotions or create a state in which people feel more indifferent to their environment than they usually would. If tricyclic antidepressants share some dopamine-blocking ability, they may also produce this effect. There are also suggestions that SSRI drugs dull or numb emotions in this way. Therefore all drugs with strong psychoactive effects may temporarily obscure or dampen feelings of depression and some sorts of drug can create a neurological state in which normal emotional responses are dampened down.

Third, trials in which antidepressants are compared with placebo are likely to become unblinded. In other words, people will be able to detect whether they have been allocated to take the antidepressant or the placebo because of the drug-induced effects produced by antidepressants. For example, people taking tricyclics will become profoundly drowsy and sedated very rapidly and people taking SSRIs often notice nausea and diarrhoea. If people can improve by taking an inert placebo, what is known as the ordinary placebo effect, then people who are taking a drug that has noticeable side effects may have a stronger or 'amplified' placebo response. Conversely, people who take the placebo may realise they have been designated to take the dummy tablet because they do not experience any of the side effects they are expecting. Such people may do worse than they might do if drug treatment had not been available in the first place. So the difference between antidepressants and placebo that is detected in clinical trials may be a result of amplified placebo effects caused by unblinding. If this is right then any drug with noticeable effects might be superior to placebo in clinical trials. The range of drugs that has been tested and found to be 'effective' in depression bears this out. Stimulants, benzodiazepines, opiates, neuroleptics and other drugs have all been found to be superior to placebo or equal to standard antidepressants in some randomised studies in people with depression.

Therefore the fact that antidepressants appear to be a bit better than placebo tablets in producing improvements in depression does not indicate that they have a disease-centred effect. It does not demonstrate that they act to reverse some hypothetical physical defect underlying depression. The physical and psychological effects they induce are quite sufficient to explain the results of existing studies, which in any case show only small differences between 'real' antidepressants and placebo or dummy tablets. The benefits that some antidepressants are said to have in other conditions such as anxiety disorders, bulimia, premenstrual tension and obsessive-compulsive disorder can also be accounted for by the mechanisms outlined here.

Long-term use

There are several studies that show that if you take people whose depression has improved while they are taking antidepressants, and you randomise some of them to have their antidepressant stopped and a placebo tablet substituted for it, then the people who are transferred to placebo will have more 'relapses' of depressive symptoms. On the basis of these studies people who have had a single episode of depression are recommended to continue to take antidepressants for at least six months. People who have had recurrent episodes are recommended to take antidepressants on a long-term basis.

However, these studies suffer from the same logical flaw as the long-term studies of neuroleptics. The people who are withdrawn from the drugs will be liable to withdrawal effects and these effects may themselves be mistaken for a relapse. In addition, people who experience withdrawal effects may realise that they have been swapped onto the placebo and this may make them anxious and vulnerable. The next time they experience problems they may lapse into a state of depression because they have come to believe that they need the drug to remain well and because they realise that they have been taken off it. This situation is likely because the people who have been entered into these trials are all people who have improved on drug treatment and have wanted to continue taking it, otherwise they would have stopped it earlier. In other words they are a selected group of people who are already convinced that they need drug treatment.

Antidepressants in severe depression

It is commonly stated that antidepressants are most effective in severe cases of depression. This belief probably goes back to statements by the man credited with doing the first research on the tricyclic antidepressant imipramine, Roland Kuhn. Kuhn asserted that imipramine had its best effects in people with more severe depression, at that time known as 'endogenous' depression. However, he produced no quantitative evidence for this assertion. Subsequent research did not support his view that endogenous depression responded more to antidepressant treatment than milder forms of depression.[16]

The National Institute of Health and Clinical Excellence (NICE) review of antidepressants published in 2004 acknowledged that antidepressants may not be useful in milder conditions but it claimed that the drugs have their most marked benefits in people with more severe depression. However, NICE's own data actually found the greatest effects compared with placebo in people whose depression was in the middle range of severity, rather than in those with the most severe depression.[17] In addition, older trials show that inpatients, who usually have greater levels of depression, show a lesser response to antidepressants than outpatients.[18] On the other hand, several reviews report an association between increasing severity and antidepressant response. However, these reviews are based on studies that mainly involve outpatients, and few include inpatients or people with the most severe depression.[19,20,21]

Overall, the evidence is contradictory. Even in the reviews that find greater effects in people with severe depression, the difference in depression scores between antidepressant and placebo groups in people with the most severe depression is only around four points on the Hamilton Rating Scale. This difference is still minimal and easily attributable to sedative effects, other drug-induced effects, or amplified placebo effects.

Common adverse effects

TCAs

Tricyclic antidepressants have potentially dangerous effects on the functioning of the heart. Like neuroleptics they slow down the conduction of electrical impulses in the heart and lead to prolongation of the QT interval on the electrocardiogram (ECG). In high doses they can cause dangerous irregularities of the heartbeat known as arrythmias and overdosing on these drugs is dangerous and often fatal. Even at normal doses they may very occasionally cause sudden death due to the heart malfunctioning.[22] They also cause postural hypotension which can cause someone to collapse on standing up. It is especially dangerous in the elderly, leading to falls. Sometimes it can be directly fatal.

In common with neuroleptics, tricyclic antidepressants lower the seizure threshold and can bring on epileptic fits. They have strong 'anticholinergic effects' including dry mouth, constipation, difficulty passing urine and blurred vision. At higher doses they may cause confusion. They also cause weight gain and sexual dysfunction including impotence, loss of libido and delayed orgasm.

MAOIs

Monoamine oxidase inhibitors are not commonly used any more, which is mainly due to the fact that they have the potential to cause a dangerous increase in blood pressure when they are combined with drugs or substances that are usually inactivated by the enzyme monoamine oxidase. One such substance is the chemical called tyramine. This chemical causes an increase in blood pressure and heart rate which can be dangerous and even fatal. It is present in many types of food, including cheese (hence the reaction sometimes known as the 'cheese effect'), and people taking MAOIs therefore have to avoid these foods. Drugs such as ephedrine and amphetamine, which can have the same effect, must also be avoided. These drugs are also dangerous if combined with many other types of psychoactive drug including opiates and tricyclic antidepressants.

SSRIs and related drugs

As already noted, the majority of the body's serotonin is in the gut. Consequently the most common effects of SSRIs are digestive and reflect increased gut activity in the form of nausea, vomiting, diarrhoea and abdominal pain. The SSRIs are also associated with sexual dysfunction, especially delayed orgasm. Despite being commonly somewhat sedating, SSRI drugs appear to cause agitation in a small number of patients.

SSRIs and suicide

It has been suggested that SSRI antidepressants can cause suicidal thoughts or even drive some people to attempt to commit suicide. It has been suggested that the mechanism for this effect, if it exists, is the agitation that is occasionally caused by SSRIs. It is thought that this effect may be so distressing that some people are driven to impulsively harm themselves or to contemplate or attempt suicide. Although regulatory authorities in Britain and the United States have issued warnings about a possible relationship between SSRIs and suicidal behaviour, the issue remains controversial. The evidence is conflicting and difficult to interpret.

The first evidence of links between SSRIs and suicidal behaviour came to light in the early 1990s when several case reports were published describing patients who became suicidal while taking Prozac.[23] Because suicide and suicidal behaviour is rare, it is difficult to study and apart from reports of individual patients, it has mainly been examined by combining the results of different studies using meta-analysis. Several meta-analyses of antidepressant studies in children and adolescents show raised rates of suicidal behaviour associated with use of SSRIs.[24,25,26,27] Two meta-analyses of trials in adults indicated small increases in suicide attempts or self-harm in people on SSRIs compared with placebo,[28,29] but some did not.[30,31] Moreover, where they have been compared with other types of antidepressants, SSRIs have not been found to be any worse in terms of increasing suicidal ideation and behaviour.[32,33]

Acts of violence and hostility have also been linked to use of SSRIs. Again, quantitative evidence is difficult to find because, like suicide, extreme violence is rare. However, evidence from case reports of violent incidents, including legal reports and data from drug-monitoring agencies suggests that a link between SSRIs and violence is at least a possibility.[34] The association, if it exists, may again be attributable to the agitation or activation caused by SSRIs. On the other hand it may be due to more general effects of psychoactive drugs on emotional responses, since all psychoactive drugs make people less sensitive to their environment and the needs of the people around them.[35]

In contrast to the suggestion that SSRIs induce suicidal behaviour in some people, many commentators allege that antidepressants reduce the risk of suicide. For example, several published papers claim to show that suicide rates have declined as a result of increased use of antidepressants over recent years. However, these papers failed to acknowledge that suicide rates in many countries had been falling for a long time prior to the surge of antidepressant prescribing that occurred after the introduction of SSRIs. A recent critical examination of this literature concluded that there was no evidence that suicide rates were falling as a consequence of antidepressant prescribing patterns.[36]

Therefore, it is difficult to demonstrate conclusively that SSRIs or any other class of antidepressant either increase or decrease suicide or suicidal behaviour. The evidence suggesting that SSRIs increase the risk of suicidal behaviour is strongest in children but it is difficult to think why effects in children would be qualitatively different from effects in adults. Given the serious nature of the events, it seems prudent to assume that there might be an increased risk of suicidal or violent behaviour with antidepressant drugs, until or unless it is proven otherwise.

Are antidepressants useful?

The first issue we need to consider when we are thinking about whether 'antidepressant' drugs have any useful effects is what exactly do we mean by depression. Of course people have always felt miserable from time to time, and some people have had episodes of very profound melancholy. But the idea that there is a common problem called 'depression' is a recent one. In fact this idea only emerged in the 1960s alongside the antidepressant drugs that were promoted to treat it.[37] Nowadays someone receives a diagnosis of depression if they fulfil the criteria laid down in diagnostic manuals, such as the *Diagnostic and Statistical Manual* (DSM), produced by the American Psychiatric Association. These manuals have shaped the modern process of psychiatric 'diagnosis'. But the people who receive this label have such a variety of problems that they really have little in common, other than the fact that they are asking for help in a certain way. In other words, they have chosen to discuss their difficulties with their doctor, rather than with a friend, a therapist or a priest.

There is not the space here to discuss in full the merits or otherwise of the concept of depression, but it is important to say here that the term 'depression' as currently used is misleading. When you say that someone has depression, you imply that they have a certain well-defined condition. You imply that they have the same thing as someone else who has depression and that the thing can be described in its own terms regardless of the situation of the person who feels it. But it has not been shown that this is a useful or meaningful way to think about our emotional states. In addition, there is no scientific evidence to support the idea that there are particular features of the brain that give rise to the particular feeling of depression. Each individual labelled as 'depressed' is struggling with their own unique difficulties. Labelling them with the pseudo-medical diagnosis of 'depression' obscures what is actually important in understanding their situation and helping them to overcome their problems.

I have argued that there is no evidence to support the view that antidepressant drugs act in a disease-centred way. In other words there is no evidence that they correct partially or wholly any part of an underlying biological abnormality. I have also suggested that a drug-centred view can account for the modest degree of superiority that antidepressants show over placebo in clinical trials. In other words the fact that antidepressants have noticeable effects such as sedation may boost the improvements ratings on depression measurement scales.

So if we accept a drug-centred account, what implications does this have for the role of drug treatment in depression? According to a drug-centred theory drugs produce drug-induced states. They do not correct underlying diseases. So the question is: Are there any drug-induced states that might be useful in depression? We know that some drugs like alcohol, opiates, cannabis and benzodiazepines produce euphoria. In other words the state of intoxication they produce is experienced as pleasant. You could argue that it might be useful to go out and have a drink occasionally if you feel depressed, to experience a temporary feeling of drug-induced pleasure, which may distract you from your troubles. However, this is unlikely to help you in the long term. The body manages to counteract the pleasure-inducing effects of these drugs if they are taken on a continuous basis. Some recreational drug users take drugs like these to avoid confronting difficult situations or painful memories, but they find they become dependent on the drugs, and experience withdrawal symptoms if they try and stop them.

Drugs that have sedative effects might be useful for insomnia, or to reduce anxiety and agitation in people said to have depression. Tricyclic antidepressants are strongly sedative and GPs probably often prescribe them at lower than recommended doses for their sedative effects. However, given the tricyclics' toxic effect on the heart, it would be safer to prescribe other sedatives such as benzodiazepines. It is difficult to see that SSRIs or other newer antidepressants have any role to play in the treatment of depression from a drug-centred perspective. They seem to have only mild psychoactive effects, and we are not certain what they consist of.

In general it seems unlikely that any drug-induced state will help someone overcome a period of misery or despair. Indeed it seems more likely that being under the influence of a mind-altering substance for a prolonged period is likely to hamper the efforts people need to make to recover from their problems. If the drug-centred model of drug action was explained to people when they were offered drug treatment to deal with their difficulties, it seems unlikely that many people would choose to take it. Many people have come to believe that their emotional life is governed by spontaneous fluctuations in their brain chemistry, and that antidepressant drugs can help put this right. If, in contrast, people were told that drug treatment would make them feel so groggy and unpleasant that they would be likely to forget their feelings for while, it seems likely that most people would find other ways to cope with their difficulties.

Chapter 6
Lithium and other drugs used for manic depression

In this chapter I will examine the evidence for the usefulness of drugs that are prescribed for manic depression, now often referred to as 'bipolar disorder'. Manic depression is a condition that has been recognised for a long time, consisting of episodes of extreme arousal, hyperactivity and elation, known as mania, often followed by episodes of severe depression. Classical manic depression is rare. It affects around 10 people per million per year.[1] However, over the last few decades, the idea has been popularised that there are less severe forms of the disorder and the concept of bipolar disorder has become malleable. Recent papers claim that up to 20% of the population may suffer from some sort of 'bipolar spectrum' disorder.[2] Alongside these changing notions of the condition of manic depression, and most likely as a cause of them, have come an increasing range of drug treatments aimed at people with 'bipolar disorders' or with difficulty controlling their emotions.

These drug treatments have recently become known as 'mood stabilisers'. The concept of the mood stabiliser appeared in the 1990s at about the time that Abbott Laboratories started marketing their version of an old epilepsy drug, sodium valproate, for the treatment of manic depression.[3] The term is generally used to refer to drugs that are prescribed to people diagnosed as having manic depression. But the implication that they stabilise mood has allowed these drugs to be prescribed to a much wider proportion of psychiatric patients. Almost by definition, people with psychiatric problems exhibit emotional turmoil from time to time. Since the invention of the concept of the mood stabiliser, such signs of emotion are interpreted as a pathological or abnormal instability of mood, and used as the justification for prescription of one of an increasing number of 'mood-stabilising' drugs. Hence, a large proportion of patients who attend psychiatric services are now prescribed one of these drugs, and drug companies are queuing up to get their drugs into this niche in the market.

However, contrary to the implication of the term 'mood stabiliser', there is no evidence that any of these drugs, or any other drugs for that matter, help to normalise emotional responses, or stabilise mood. From a drug-centred perspective, all drugs currently designated as 'mood stabilisers' have sedative effects and hence they are likely to suppress or flatten emotional reactions in general. The main research that has been conducted into their effects on people with psychiatric disorders, and that is used to justify the term 'mood stabiliser', concerns whether or not they suppress signs of mania and prevent relapse in people diagnosed with classical manic depression, otherwise known as 'bipolar I disorder'. The only tests that have been done to look at how these drugs affect the variability of mood in healthy volunteers were done with lithium, and found that lithium did not reduce normal fluctuations of mood.[4,5]

The history of lithium

The first drug that was regarded as a specific treatment for manic depression was lithium. The fact that lithium became established as a psychiatric treatment is one of the more bizarre episodes in the history of psychopharmacology. Lithium is a toxic alkali metal, in the same class as sodium and potassium. It was used as a treatment for gout throughout the nineteenth century and despite the fact that it was found to be ineffective in this condition, it continued to be used well into the twentieth century. This meant that lithium was present in hospital pharmacies in the 1950s. John Cade, an Australian psychiatrist, started experimenting with the use of lithium in the late 1940s. He injected guinea pigs with it and observed that they became sedated. From this observation he deduced that it might be useful in mania and he tried it out on ten patients with long-term mania and some patients with schizophrenia. He published the results of this experiment in 1949, claiming that lithium had achieved remarkable results, particularly in the patients with mania. His claims were taken up by a small group of European researchers who championed the use of lithium until it was accepted as a standard psychiatric treatment. However, this might never have been achieved if lithium had not previously been used as a medical treatment. The fact that it had been widely used for gout and other complaints such as arthritis and kidney stones meant that there was a precedent for using lithium as a medical drug. It did not seem unusual therefore to use this toxic metal as a form of treatment. In addition, it meant that there was a supply of lithium in hospital pharmacies ready to administer to people admitted with manic-depressive episodes. John Cade experimented with other toxic elements such as caesium and strontium for the treatment of psychiatric disorders, but unsurprisingly these were never adopted. It also turned out that Cade had 'sexed' up the results of his lithium trial. Looking at the notes Cade made during the trial, historian Neil Johnson revealed that it was generally difficult to distinguish between toxic and 'therapeutic' effects and many incidents of lithium toxicity had not been reported in the published paper.

Drug-induced effects of lithium and other mood stabilisers

Lithium is a metal that causes severe damage to the nervous system, the gut and the kidneys at relatively low doses. Mild symptoms of toxicity include neurological symptoms such as tremor and lethargy. Progressive damage results in diarrhoea and vomiting, incontinence, drowsiness, disorientation, abnormal jerking movements, loss of balance (ataxia) and slurred speech (dysarthria), finally giving rise to convulsions, coma and death. The so-called therapeutic effects are on a continuum with the manifestations of the toxic state. Thus before the signs of full-blown toxicity start, lithium causes suppression of nervous conduction leading to sedation and impairment of mental functioning. These effects are clearly demonstrated in volunteer studies.[6,7] After two to three weeks on lithium volunteers show decreased ability to learn new information, prolonged reaction times, poor memory, loss of interest and reduced spontaneous activity. Therefore it is not surprising that people with mania and other forms of over-arousal are subdued when given lithium. The trouble is, because it is so toxic, the doses required to achieve a useful sedative effect are perilously close to those that cause a dangerous toxic state. This is why patients on lithium have to have their blood lithium levels monitored on a regular basis.

Other drugs now referred to as 'mood stabilisers' are all sedative drugs that suppress nervous activity in different ways. They all cause drowsiness at normal therapeutic doses and the anticonvulsant drugs cause signs of nervous toxicity such as slurred speech (dysarthria) and loss of balance (ataxia) at high doses and sometimes also at lower doses.

The specificity of lithium

Although lithium is still recommended for the treatment of acute mania, in practice it is rarely used alone for this purpose. This is because its toxic potential prevents an adequate sedative effect from being achieved. Therefore neuroleptics and benzodiazepines, and more recently the anti-epileptic sedative drug sodium valproate, are the mainstay of treatment. Lithium is now mainly associated with the long-term treatment of manic depression, where it is believed to reduce the risk of recurrence of a further episode. Although there is no biochemical theory, such as the dopamine hypothesis of schizophrenia, that helps to rationalise a disease-centred view of the action of lithium in this circumstance, it is clear that lithium is not simply regarded as a sedative. If it was, the risk of its toxic effects could surely not be justified. Instead lithium is regarded as having a specific, although as yet unidentified, action on the presumed biological basis of abnormal mood or manic depression.

However, there is little evidence that lithium is actually better than other sorts of drugs with sedative effects for treating people with manic depression. In fact two studies of drug treatment for people with acute mania found that lithium was inferior to neuroleptics, probably due to the limitations caused by its toxicity.[8,9] The authors of one of these studies described how the most severely disturbed patients who were randomised to lithium had to be placed in secluded, locked rooms in order to keep them in the study.[10] In contrast a Japanese study found lithium to be superior. However, doses of lithium were four times those of chlorpromazine and patients were less severely ill, and therefore probably did not require the same level of sedation as patients in the other studies .[11]

Two studies have examined whether people with a diagnosis of mania do better with lithium compared to people with a diagnosis of another acute psychotic disorder, such as acute schizophrenia. Both of these studies compared lithium with a neuroleptic drug and found that diagnosis did not predict which drug treatment people responded to. In other words, people with mania responded just as well to the neuroleptic drug as they did to lithium and people with acute schizophrenia responded just as well to lithium.[12,13] One of these studies claimed that mood-related symptoms responded better to lithium and positive symptoms of schizophrenia responded better to neuroleptics. However, a tortuous statistical analysis was required to demonstrate this point, and the graphs provided in the published paper do not show a convincing picture.[14] In contrast, one of the earlier comparisons of neuroleptics and lithium found that the neuroleptic was superior or equivalent to lithium for many typical manic symptoms.[15]

There has been little research into the effects of benzodiazepines in mania, despite the fact that they are widely used in this disorder. Since they are sedative drugs, and mania is a condition of increased arousal, benzodiazepines would be a logical intervention and target for research. Some small studies that compared a benzodiazepine called clonazepam with lithium reported that the clonazepam was superior, but these were never followed up.[16,17] Whether this means that the results did not fulfil their early promise or whether the drug company that conducted them decided to aim the drug at a different market is uncertain.

No research has attempted to establish the specificity of other drugs used as treatments for manic depression. Many atypical neuroleptics are now being used for the treatment of mania. The fact that all have been shown to have similar efficacy compared with placebo is further evidence that, as would be expected, any drug with a sedative action exerts a therapeutic effect in mania.[18]

Evidence on the long-term effects of lithium and other mood stabilisers

The widest use of lithium and other mood stabilisers is for the long-term treatment of people with manic depression. Guidelines suggest that they should be prescribed on a long-term basis to someone with this diagnosis in order to reduce the risk of relapse into an episode of either mania or depression. These recommendations are based on placebo-controlled trials, some of which show that people taking a mood stabiliser relapse less frequently than people taking placebo. However, these trials suffer from the same problems as the trials of long-term neuroleptic treatment. They are mostly discontinuation studies. In other words, people who are already taking medication are randomised to continue to take it or to have a placebo substituted for their active drugs. Therefore people who take placebo are actually people who have just had their previous long-term medication withdrawn.

There is strong evidence that discontinuing lithium can induce a relapse in someone with manic depression, especially a relapse of mania. There is even evidence to show that the likelihood of having a relapse after you stop long-term lithium is higher than it is before lithium is started.[19] The early studies of lithium, which were conducted in the 1970s, mostly involved people who were taking lithium prior to the study. Three further studies have been carried out since 1990. In these studies at least 20–30% of subjects had been on lithium prior to entering the study. One of these studies found no difference between lithium and placebo.[20] One found a difference, but it was clinically small.[21] Another reported a more substantial difference, but it appears that a large proportion of patients (up to 69%) may have been taking lithium prior to the study, although the published paper does not make this clear.[22] The majority of the difference in relapse rates concerned manic relapses, which occurred early on in the study. This supports the possibility that the study demonstrates a discontinuation effect, since patients on placebo are likely to suffer the consequences of lithium withdrawal more strongly immediately after they are placed on placebo, during the early part of the trial.

None of these recent studies took the discontinuation effect into account, despite the fact that it is now widely accepted that lithium discontinuation can induce relapse. It would have been relatively easy to look at results for people who had not been on lithium for some time prior to the study, for example, or to use statistical techniques to examine the impact of having been taken off lithium. Therefore, like the situation with the neuroleptics, the research into the prophylactic effects of long-term lithium only shows that stopping lithium, once it is started, increases the risk of having a relapse. No research has yet managed to establish whether starting lithium in the first place has any beneficial effects in terms of reducing relapse rates.

The evidence is just as poor for other 'mood stabilisers', if not worse. The only long-term study of sodium valproate versus placebo and lithium found no difference between any of the treatments on any of the major outcome measures.[23] Lamotrigine, a relatively new 'mood stabiliser', was found to be better than placebo for preventing depressive episodes in two trials sponsored by the manufacturer.[24,25] However, as explained in the previous chapter, there are manifold drug-centred explanations for why drugs might appear to be better than an inert placebo in depression, so it is not possible to conclude that lamotrigine has a specific therapeutic effect. There is one placebo-controlled trial of olanzapine for the prophylaxis of manic depression.[26] Again the results indicate a probable discontinuation effect in the placebo group, since the majority of the relapses in the placebo group occurred in the first three weeks of the study and all had occurred by three months. This is highly suggestive that relapses were either induced by discontinuation of olanzapine, which all participants were taking prior to randomisation, or that withdrawal symptoms were mistaken for relapse in people who were placed on placebo.

Adverse effects

Mood stabilisers now comprise a diverse group of drugs with different pharmacological actions. Therefore their adverse effects vary.

Lithium is highly toxic to the nervous system, the digestive system and the kidneys. This means that blood levels that are only slightly higher than the levels usually associated with current doses can cause an acute toxic state that rapidly results in death if the lithium is not stopped immediately. This dangerous toxic state can occur if an overdose of lithium is taken, but it also occurs if blood levels increase slightly because of dehydration or interactions with other drugs. The toxic state can also sometimes occur at what would normally be regarded as safe blood levels of lithium.[27] Before the full-blown toxic state develops, lithium's effects on the kidneys result in extreme thirst and excessive urination. In a small proportion of patients, long-term treatment may result in irreversible kidney damage.[28] Its effects on the nervous system commonly result in a hand tremor as well as reduced reaction times, slow thinking and reduced creativity.[29] Lithium also frequently results in under-activity of the thyroid gland. Up to 20% of women on long-term treatment develop this complication and require treatment with thyroid hormones.[30] It is usually reversible on stopping lithium. Lithium can also affect the parathyroid gland, which affects calcium levels and bones. Lithium frequently causes weight gain.

Valproic acid, brand name Depakote, is essentially the same drug as sodium valproate, a drug that has been used in the treatment of epilepsy for many years. This drug is known to cause liver failure in a small minority of children who take it and it has other dangerous but rare complications including pancreatitis, which can be fatal, and blood disorders, such as thrombocytopaenia (suppression of platelets, the blood cells involved in clotting) and pancytopaenia (suppression of all blood cells). More commonly it causes nausea, lethargy and sedation, hair loss, weight gain and polycystic ovaries, a condition associated with reduced fertility. It is also known to produce a high rate of foetal abnormalities if it is taken early in pregnancy. Drugs that cause foetal malformations do so in the early weeks of pregnancy, often before the woman knows that she is pregnant. Therefore it is often not possible to stop the drug before the damage is done. For this reason, as well as the fact that it is likely to impair fertility, many people suggest that it should not be prescribed to women of childbearing age, but frequently is.

Carbamezepine is another anti-epileptic drug that has become popular as a 'mood stabiliser'. It also causes a rash, nausea, sedation and signs of neurotoxicity such as loss of balance (ataxia) and double vision (diploplia). It can also cause serious blood disorders, such as aplastic anaemia and agranulocytosis, by suppressing the production of blood cells in the bone marrow. Very rarely it causes a drug-induced reaction known as 'hypersensitivity syndrome', a dangerous condition which can lead to failure of internal organs, especially the liver, and has a death rate of 8%. It can also cause a serious skin reaction (toxic epidermal necrolysis).

Lamotrigine is a relatively new anti-epileptic drug. It also causes neurological symptoms such as ataxia and diploplia. It can cause a rash, vomiting and it too may impair liver function. It has also been associated with blood disorders and with the drug hypersensitivity syndrome.

Pros and cons of drug use in manic depression or bipolar disorder

Sedative drugs of any sort appear to be helpful in suppressing the manifestations of acute mania. We know that mania is self-limiting, that is it will eventually subside, but while it lasts it can be devastating. Therefore the use of sedative drugs may be helpful while the underlying disturbance runs its course. Recommended drugs are neuroleptics, lithium and various anticonvulsants, but as mentioned earlier, benzodiazepines are used liberally in conjunction with all of these. Since benzodiazepines are less unpleasant and probably less harmful than recommended treatments, it would be useful to have more research into their use. Research into whether they could be used on their own for the treatment of mania would be particularly helpful. The main problem with the use of benzodiazepines is likely to be the development of tolerance to their effects, leading to the need for higher and higher doses.

The evidence presented so far suggests that we cannot be certain that any drug genuinely helps people with manic depression in the long term, in terms of reducing the risk of having a further episode. From a drug-centred perspective, it is plausible that sedative drugs might suppress the occurrence of mania, since it is a state of increased arousal. However, it is also possible that the body's adaptations to the long-term use of a drug will counteract any suppressant effect the drug might initially exert. It is difficult to see how the use of sedative and deactivating drugs like lithium, neuroleptics and anti-epileptic drugs can prevent the occurrence of depression. Indeed, according to a drug-centred model, these sorts of drugs would be more likely to induce the occurrence of depression or a depression-like state.

For people with manic depression the question is whether to endure the unpleasant and sometimes dangerous effects of the various drugs commonly on offer, for the hope of a possible reduction of the risk of relapse. Manic depression is a frightening condition, which can wreck people's families and jobs and leave people with devastating debts and other problems. Some people may feel that even the hope of a small effect may compensate for all the unpleasant and adverse effects of long-term drug treatment. However, some will prefer to find other ways to try and exert some control over their condition. For example, some people manage to identify the early warning signs of mania and can use sedative drugs and lifestyle measures such as avoiding stress and taking time off work, to try and avert an impending relapse. Some people may simply prefer to live with the risk of recurrence, and seek treatment and support if and when they need it.

People who do not have classical manic depression need to know that there is no evidence to support the use of a so-called mood stabiliser. No drugs have been shown to normalise or smooth out moods, and all drugs prescribed as mood stabilisers are sedative drugs of one form or another. These drugs suppress mental and physical activity and probably reduce people's emotional responses to their environment, in a similar way to neuroleptics. Again, some people may decide that such an effect is useful to help them manage a period of emotional crisis. However, people need to be aware that rather than rectifying an abnormal brain state, the drugs produce a global state of mental suppression. It seems unlikely that many people would feel that pharmacological restriction of this sort was useful or desirable in the long term.

Chapter 7
Stimulants

Stimulants are a group of drugs that are still referred to by the type of effect they induce rather than the condition for which they are prescribed. They are controlled drugs and some, such as amphetamine and cocaine, are commonly used as recreational drugs. In fact all drugs classed as stimulants have the potential to be abused. The main indication for which stimulants are prescribed is a set of behavioural problems in children that used to be called hyperactivity disorder and is now known as attention deficit hyperactivity disorder or ADHD. The stimulant methylphenidate, trade name Ritalin, is most commonly prescribed, but various forms of amphetamine are also used. There is also a growing trend to diagnose and treat ADHD in adults, again using stimulants as the main form of treatment.

What effects do stimulants produce?

Although popular literature suggests that stimulants correct a chemical imbalance, there is no evidence of a specific chemical imbalance in the brains of people with attention deficit disorder, and no evidence that stimulants work in this way. Some accounts suggest that an abnormality of the dopamine system has been shown. Research into dopamine has been conducted because stimulants are known to affect the dopamine system. In contrast to the neuroleptics, stimulants increase the availability and activity of dopamine. A few studies have suggested there might be an abnormality of the protein that transports dopamine out of the gap between the nerve terminals.[1] However, as with the studies of dopamine in schizophrenia or psychosis, there was no attempt in these studies to control for other factors that are known to influence dopamine activity, such as anxiety, stress and movement and only a few mentioned smoking and use of drugs other than stimulants. In addition, the studies were small, and most involved some subjects who had already been treated with stimulants or other drugs known to effect dopamine transmission.

In fact, as with neuroleptics, there is no need to construct a disease-centred account for the action of stimulants. A drug-centred model can easily account for their effects in ADHD. The features of mild stimulant-induced intoxication are likely to have impressive effects on hyperactivity and concentration. These effects have been shown to occur in all children and adults, regardless of whether they have been diagnosed with ADHD or not.[2]

The main physiological effect of stimulant drugs is to increase arousal. At high doses this results in increased activity and it can cause obsessive-compulsive behaviours and abnormal movements such as tics and grimaces, which have been recognised for many years in the drug-using community. However, at lower doses the main manifestation of increased arousal is an increased ability to concentrate, and a feeling of calm. This is familiar to people who smoke cigarettes, since nicotine is a mild stimulant drug. Therefore it should not be surprising that stimulants improve attention and reduce hyperactivity in the relatively low doses at which they are prescribed. However, there is more to this effect. Animal studies show that stimulants inhibit spontaneous exploratory behaviour, reduce an animal's interest in its environment and reduce its social interactions with other animals. In the place of these normal interactive behaviours the animal shows repetitive, over-focused, pointless behaviours such as pacing, scratching, excessive grooming, gnawing and staring at small objects. They also develop tics and other involuntary abnormal movements.[3] Therefore it appears that stimulants increase the ability of a person or an animal to focus on a single task by reducing their interaction with the rest of the environment.

In children too it is recognised that stimulants can suppress interest, spontaneity and emotional responsiveness. This effect is sometimes referred to as a 'zombie-like' state. In most psychiatric literature these effects are reported as the mental 'side effects' of treatment but their relation to the more desirable effects is obvious. These effects are well described in a report of an early controlled trial of Ritalin:

> [The children became] distinctly more bland or 'flat' emotionally, lacking both the age-typical variety and frequency of emotional expression. They responded less, exhibited little or no initiative and spontaneity, offered little indication of either interest or aversion, showed virtually no curiosity, surprise, or pleasure, and seemed devoid of humor. Jocular comments and humorous situations passed unnoticed. In short, while on active drug treatment, the children were relatively but unmistakeably affectless, humorless, and apathetic.[4]

Children themselves do not like the experience of being on stimulants. In interviews and feedback they reveal that they feel unhappy and wish to be like they were before they started.[5] One study of children's views on their medication found that although children rarely complained about medication to their doctors, there was 'a pervasive dislike among hyperactive children for taking stimulants'. Verbatim comments from the children interviewed for this study described the experience of taking stimulants in the following ways: the drug 'numbed me', 'It makes me sad', 'I wouldn't smile or anything', 'It takes over of me', 'Don't feel like myself'.[6]

In many cases prescribed stimulants produce effects typically associated with recreational use or misuse. They commonly produce insomnia, for example, they may cause agitation and occasionally, with continual use, they can drive people into psychosis. As already mentioned they cause abnormal movements such as twitches and tics. In two prevalence studies 8–9% of children taking stimulants developed tics or other abnormal movements.[7,8]

When stimulants are used recreationally, people often have to increase the dose to keep getting the effect or the 'buzz' that they want to experience. This shows that stimulants, like other psychoactive drugs, induce 'tolerance'. In other words the body adapts to counteract their effects, so if you use them continuously, you have to increase the dose to get the same effects. Tolerance to stimulants prescribed for ADHD has been demonstrated in animals[9] and documented in children.[10] Predictably, there is little information about how common and profound this effect is. In theory, however, tolerance may obliterate any beneficial effects that are experienced in the early days of stimulant treatment. Alternatively, ever-increasing doses may be required to obtain the effect that was initially observed.

Although stimulants do not result in the severe and sometimes dangerous withdrawal syndromes associated with drugs like alcohol and heroin, it is now recognised that when someone stops taking stimulants they will experience withdrawal symptoms. Long-term drug abusers experience fatigue, lethargy and depression, sometimes accompanied by suicidal ideation after withdrawal. People can also become anxious and irritable, memory is impaired and after an initial period of insomnia, sleep is increased in reaction to the prolonged arousal and insomnia induced by the drugs. Children who stop prescribed stimulants may experience a 'rebound' phenomenon. This is when they become more hyperactive and disturbed than they were before taking the drug. It may be similar to the anxiety and restlessness produced by nicotine withdrawal.

Evidence for their usefulness

Several randomised trials have shown that over a few days or weeks, stimulant drugs improve attention and hyperactivity better than a placebo. It is particularly these symptoms that are improved. Stimulants do not appear to be superior to a placebo for the other problems that such children often have, for example impulsive behaviour, poor social skills or aggression. However, a review of these placebo-controlled studies conducted by the respected Cochrane Collaboration (an international network of medical experts who summarise and analyse research on medical interventions) noted that most of the studies were of poor quality and there was evidence of publication bias. In other words it is likely that there are additional unpublished studies that show no difference between stimulants and placebo. Only nine trials were identified that lasted for longer than four weeks. The longest lasted for 28 weeks (approximately six months).[11] Bear in mind that most of the time stimulants are prescribed for years at a time. These trials provided no evidence that there was a true benefit from taking stimulants over longer durations.

Recently a large long-term multicentre randomised trial was conducted comparing four groups of patients: one had intensive behavioural therapy; one had an intensive 'medication management' regime involving frequent reviews with a doctor; one had a combination of behavioural therapy and medication management; and one received routine community care. This last option often involved receiving medication. This study, the Multimodal Treatment Study of Children with ADHD, or the MTA study, has been presented as definitively establishing the superiority of stimulant medication for the treatment of ADHD. Some psychiatrists have even argued that medication should now be the sole form of treatment for ADHD and that psychosocial interventions are pointless. But the story is a little more complex. The study involved a total of 579 children and treatment lasted for 14 months. The first set of results, based on data from the 14 months of the study, showed that all groups showed a substantial decline in the severity of their symptoms. The medication management group fared better than the group that had behaviour therapy on the core symptoms of inattention, as rated by parents and teachers, and hyperactivity as rated by parents only. It is this finding that has been highlighted. However, most of the people doing the outcome ratings were not blinded, so expectation or placebo effects may have influenced outcome. The ratings by the only blinded rater, a classroom observer, showed no difference between the treatment groups for any measures, including attention or hyperactivity.[12] In addition, around 60% of the routine community treatment group also received medication and this group fared the same as the behavioural therapy group. Hence it appears that there was something about the intensity of the contact involved in the intensive medication management group that improved symptoms and the superior outcome of this group cannot simply be attributed to drug therapy. Another problem that has been overlooked is that around a quarter to a third of children had been using stimulants prior to the study. Hence some children assigned to behavioural therapy would have had their medication stopped at the beginning of the study. These children may have suffered from withdrawal effects that may have been mistaken for symptoms. The study showed no differences between the different treatment groups for the other factors that were evaluated including aggression, social skills, parent–child relations and academic achievement.

The three-year follow-up of the MTA study was published in 2007. After 14 months subjects were free to seek whatever treatment regime they desired. The proportion of subjects in the behavioural treatment group who took medication increased, and the proportion in the medication management group reduced. However, 71% of subjects in the medication group took medication most of the time versus only 45% in the group that originally received behaviour therapy. The proportion in the routine treatment group was unchanged. The results showed that there was no difference between the original groups in terms of any outcome measures at three years.[13] Convinced supporters of stimulants may wonder whether this negative result was due to the fact that the differences in the numbers of subjects taking medications in the different groups had decreased. That is, more children in the behavioural therapy group were taking stimulants during the later part of the follow-up period, and some children in the medication management group stopped taking drugs. However, another analysis showed that there was also no difference on any outcome measures between children who had consistently taken medication over the whole three-year period, children who had taken medication inconsistently and children who had not taken medication at all. The lack of superiority of drug treatment could not be explained by children who took medication having more severe symptoms, since the severity of the symptoms at the start of the study was the same for children who used medication continuously, intermittently and not at all.[14]

So although it has been shown that stimulants improve attention and reduce activity levels in the short term, there is no good evidence that these effects persist with long-term use. The MTA study indicated that stimulants might have been modestly superior to behaviour therapy at 14 months for reducing hyperactivity and improving attention. However, as I have pointed out, the only double-blind ratings made in this study did not confirm this finding. After three years any advantage for stimulant treatment had definitely been lost. In addition, even the initial 14-month assessment failed to indicate any beneficial effects on school performance or family relations.

Harmful consequences of their use

Stimulants are often said to be very safe drugs and they have been used for many decades. However, they do have a number of well-recognised and worrying adverse effects. The most important of these is that they suppress growth. Although this has been shown in studies going back to the 1970s, it has been played down in official literature, and some important researchers with extensive links to the pharmaceutical industry have challenged whether it exists at all. These researchers have suggested that it is the disorder of ADHD itself that retards growth, rather than the medication.[15] However, data from the MTA study makes the link between stimulants and reduced growth difficult to dispute. At the three-year follow-up of the MTA study, children who had taken medication on a continuous basis were 2.3cm smaller than a non-ADHD comparison group and an enormous 4.2cm shorter than those children in the study who had not used stimulants.[16] Children who had started stimulants for the first time at the beginning of the study, that is children who had not been taking them prior to entering the study, were 3cm shorter than children in the study who did not take medication and 1.1cm shorter than the non-ADHD comparison group. Although not all studies show negative effects on growth, another recent study looking at growth rates over five years confirmed the MTA findings and showed that higher doses of stimulants had a stronger retarding effect on growth than lower doses.[17] This data suggests there is a considerable loss of growth over a three-year period. However, the Royal College of Psychiatrists' information leaflet about stimulants, published in 2004, does not even mention growth reduction under its list of 'side effects'. It only states that 'because of the effect on appetite, the child's height and weight should be measured regularly'.[18]

The exact mechanism whereby stimulants suppress growth is not yet known. It may be related to the fact that they reduce appetite, but they are also known to have an impact on several hormones that may be involved in growth including growth hormone, prolactin and thyroid hormones.

Growth suppression may not just effect height.[19] If the body's growth is slowed down, the body's internal organs, including the brain, are also likely to show impaired growth and this has been demonstrated in one animal study.[20] In addition, stimulant use may interfere with the process of puberty. The hormones involved in growth are also involved in sexual maturation. Surprisingly, there is almost no research into the effects of methylphenidate on the process of puberty, even though many millions of children and adolescents are placed on these drugs through this period of their development. Similarly, although it is often stated that growth suppression does not affect ultimate height, I could only locate one study that actually looked at this.[21] This study did not detect any difference between the height of 61 17-year-olds previously diagnosed with ADHD and treated with stimulants for at least six months, and 99 control boys of the same age who did not have ADHD.

One of the ways the impact of stimulants on growth has been minimised is through the suggestion that 'rebound' growth can occur after stimulants are stopped. In other words, the body grows faster than usual after stopping stimulants to make up for the reduced pace of growth induced by the drugs. Some evidence suggests this does occur, although it is not certain whether this phenomenon is able to make up for the loss of growth that occurs while on stimulants, especially if they are taken for many years. In addition, unnaturally fast growth spurts may also have adverse consequences, and cannot simply be assumed to undo the damage done by the drugs.

Stimulant drugs increase the activity of the heart. This is manifested in an increase in the heart rate and blood pressure. Drug abusers who are heavy users of cocaine or amphetamines are known to have a higher than normal risk of heart disease, including sudden death due to heart attacks and heart failure. In 2006 a series of cases of sudden death in children taking stimulants for ADHD was reported to the American drug regulator, the FDA (Food and Drug Administration). Some, but not all of the children, were found to have had structural abnormalities of the heart that were present from birth. In these cases the heart was already compromised and could not cope with the extra demands placed on it by the stimulant drugs. However, some cases occurred in children with apparently normal hearts. The FDA subsequently issued a warning about the possibility that stimulants might cause sudden death in children. Proponents of stimulant treatment argued against this warning, claiming that the risks of stimulants had been exaggerated. A consultant to the FDA committee that issued the warning responded that cases of sudden death linked to stimulants were likely to be greater than the number reported and that 'increasing heart rate and blood pressure by the administration of powerful cardiac stimulants is inherently risky' (p. 2296).[22,23]

It is well established that increases in heart rate and blood pressure increase the risk of heart attacks and strokes in adults. Adults who take stimulants should be aware that they are likely to increase their risk of suffering the consequences of heart disease.

Stimulants are well known to cause psychosis if taken at high doses for long periods. Some people are more susceptible to this effect than others, and hence it does occasionally occur in children who take prescribed doses of Ritalin and other stimulants.

As described above, the use of stimulants can have other more subtle adverse mental effects. In some cases they induce a depressive picture, with lethargy, withdrawal, and loss of emotional responsiveness. In others they may cause agitation and anxiety. Insomnia is very common.

Another common problem with stimulant use is the 'rebound' phenomenon. Most stimulant drugs are short acting, and are eliminated from the body rapidly. When the effects of the drug wear off, the child starts to show all the behaviours that were suppressed by the drug, but often with even greater intensity than before as a reaction to the previous suppression. This appears to confirm to the child, their parents and teachers that the stimulants are really helping, and it may be necessary to give the child further doses to calm their behaviour. However, this rebound state is likely to be an acute withdrawal state. In other words it is simply the body's reaction to having the drug removed which may make the child's behaviour worse than it was before taking the treatment. Similarly, when long-term drug treatment is stopped, the return of disruptive behaviours is likely to be interpreted as the re-emergence of the underlying symptoms, and taken as confirmation that continued treatment is necessary. However, as with other psychiatric drugs, behaviour following the cessation of treatment is likely to be caused at least in part by the body's reaction to the withdrawal of the drug and it may have nothing to do with the original problem. Both these phenomena mean that it may be difficult for children or adults to stop taking stimulants once they have started.

The relation between prescribed stimulants and drug abuse

There has been some controversy about whether the prescription of stimulant drugs for childhood disorders might increase the abuse of stimulants and other drugs in later life. All the stimulant medications that are prescribed are known to be abused, including Ritalin. Some children are known to sell their prescribed medication to other children or young people for recreational use. It is also known that children who are diagnosed with ADHD have higher rates of substance abuse subsequently compared with children without a psychiatric diagnosis.[24] The conventional wisdom is that taking stimulants does not add further to this risk, and may reduce the likelihood of someone with ADHD developing substance-abuse problems later on. A meta-analysis of six studies conducted in 2003 found that there was an overall reduction in substance abuse among people treated with stimulants compared to those who were not.[25] However, these studies suffered from problems such as following children up too young, before many of them had been exposed to illicit drugs, and looking only at occasional rather than problematic use of substances. In addition, some of the studies appeared to involve atypical samples of children. For example, in one of the studies the ADHD children who were not taking stimulant medication were much more severely disturbed on a whole range of parameters than those who were. In general the opposite would be expected, since medication is generally still reserved for those in the more severe symptom range. Hence in this sample it is likely that rates of substance abuse were higher than they would be in a more usual group of non-medicated children.[26] If the sample had been more typical, the results may have been different.

One large and well-conducted study followed up children from childhood through to an average age of 26. This study found that children who were diagnosed with ADHD had higher rates of smoking and substance abuse in adult life. In addition, a careful analysis was conducted that took into account the effects of other factors that are known to predict the development of substance abuse problems in later life, such as having parents who use drugs. This analysis found, after accounting for the effects of other predictive factors, that being prescribed stimulant medication in childhood increased the likelihood of becoming a regular smoker and of becoming dependent on stimulant drugs such as cocaine and amphetamine.[27]

The three-year follow up of the MTA study found that 13% of children randomised to behaviour therapy had used illicit substances compared with 22% of children randomised to medication management.[28] Although the difference is not tested in the paper, I conducted a statistical test which showed this difference may not simply be due to chance.[29] The analysis presented in the paper, which rightly controlled for the effects of other factors that may predict later behavioural problems, found that children who took prescribed medication for more days during the follow-up had statistically higher rates of delinquent behaviour than other children, but not of substance use.

Deciding whether to use stimulants

Taking stimulant medication undoubtedly has profound effects on children and adults. The drugs can reduce hyperactive behaviour and improve attention in the short term. These effects may bring relief to parents and teachers who are struggling to control a disruptive child. They may help a child who is distracted from their schoolwork through distress or through boredom to focus their attention more intensely on the tasks they are set. If a family feel they are simply not able to cope in any other way with a child's behaviour, a period of stimulant treatment may be able to provide a window of respite and opportunity. However, there is no evidence to suggest that long-term stimulant treatment ultimately benefits the child or the family.

The reasons not to use stimulants, or to limit their use to short periods only, are not just confined to their physical adverse effects. Taking regular medication of any sort for a behavioural problem conveys a strong message to children. It implies that they are not in control of their own behaviour and that they require a drug in order to be 'good', and to do well. Research on children diagnosed with ADHD shows that they accept the idea their doctor tells them that their behaviour is caused by a brain defect and that they require a drug to correct it. They draw the conclusion that they cannot exert any control over themselves. This allows them to avoid taking responsibility for 'bad' behaviour, which they can blame on their ADHD or on missing their medication. However, the other side of this view is that they don't believe they deserve any credit for their good behaviour, or for their successes. They are often frightened to come off the drugs, and have no confidence in their abilities to perform or behave well without medication.[30] Children who believe they cannot control their behaviour are likely to view themselves in a generally negative way. They become demoralised. Follow-up studies of children who have been on long-term treatment for ADHD suggest they often suffer from low self-esteem.[31] Of course this is likely to be due in part to the original problems, the problems that led to the child being diagnosed with ADHD in the first place. But it is also possible that children's experience of drug treatment further lowers their already battered view of their own worth.

These beliefs are often reinforced by the adults in the child's life. Teachers and parents often concur in the belief that bad behaviour is a result of the disease and good behaviour is the effects of the drug. Therefore, the child no longer gets the rewards and sanctions they need to enable them to master their own behaviour and mature properly.[32]

It is possible therefore that the prescription of medication for 'attention deficit disorder' will produce a generation of young people who have difficulty taking responsibility for their actions, have low self-esteem and no confidence in their ability to negotiate the pitfalls of life unaided by a chemical crutch. It would not be surprising if such people turned to drug abuse as a way of dealing with stresses or became lifelong consumers of psychiatric drugs and services.

Stimulants are powerful psychoactive drugs like the other drugs described in this book. In low doses they subdue hyperactive behaviour and increase attention by mildly increasing arousal. Anyone in a mildly hyper-aroused state will focus more intensely on a single task. In evolutionary terms a state of arousal is useful when people have to run away from a threat or attack an enemy and so need to concentrate on a specific object. In this situation it is also necessary to shut off a person's inclination to interact with the wider environment. You don't want a soldier or a hunter to be distracted by a beautiful flower. The focusing of attention is achieved therefore by suppressing people's ability to interact with other aspects of their environment, to explore, to play, to be creative. But these are the activities that constitute the very essence of childhood. They are what make children happy, and they are the activities that enable children to learn and develop.

Overall the main message is that medicating children should not be done lightly. It is essential to explore all possible alternatives for amending behaviour before drugs are prescribed. Schools, parents and mental health services need to co-operate to reduce the reliance on stimulants and to publicise alternative approaches. If stimulants are prescribed, people need to know that there is no evidence that they have any long-term benefits and that they may be difficult to stop once started. Adverse effects such as growth suppression and effects on the heart are now undeniable. The psychological impact of medicating children in order to change their behaviour may be even more worrying.

Chapter 8
Benzodiazepines

Benzodiazepine is the chemical name for a group of drugs discovered in the 1960s. The individual drugs are often more familiar by their trade names. One of the most commonly used benzodiazepines is diazepam, whose trade name is Valium. They also include chlordiazepoxide (Librium), nitrazepam (Mogadon), lorazepam (Ativan), and temazepam. Benzodiazepines are drugs with sedative properties, similar in nature to alcohol. They cause a sensation of pleasure or euphoria as well as sedation, and they are abused by drug users, especially those who have a preference for sedative drugs or 'downers'. They are often used concurrently with heroin for example and many heroin users are also addicted to benzodiazepines.

In psychiatry benzodiazepines have a wide range of uses. From the 1960s onwards they were widely prescribed to people with sleeping difficulties and people with anxiety and neurotic disorders, especially women, often for long periods of time. In the 1980s it became apparent that most people who take benzodiazepines for more than a few weeks become physically dependent on them and experience withdrawal symptoms when they stop. Recommendations were then made that they should not be prescribed routinely other than for short periods. They are still regarded as an effective treatment of anxiety disorders, but their use for this purpose has declined. Benzodiazepines are also frequently prescribed to people with severe psychiatric disorders because of their sedative properties and they are prescribed extensively to psychiatric inpatients with all sorts of diagnoses.

Benzodiazepines act by influencing the activity of the brain chemical known as GABA. GABA is found in all parts of the brain and it is the brain's main inhibitory neurotransmitter. In other words it reduces the activity of the brain. Benzodiazepines enhance the inhibitory activity of GABA. Therefore they lower the activity of the brain causing sedation and relaxation at lower doses, progressing to sleep and then coma and death at very high doses. However, they are relatively safe compared with other drugs that depress the activity of the brain and the nervous system like alcohol, barbiturates, opiates and neuroleptics. They do not have the adverse effects on the heart induced by the neuroleptics, and they usually only cause dangerous levels of sedation at very high doses.

In most situations benzodiazepines are regarded as non-specific treatments. In other words, they are thought to work according to a drug-centred model by producing a drug-induced sedative state, rather than reversing an underlying disease. Since it is well known that they induce similar effects in everyone, regardless of whether or not they suffer from a psychiatric problem, it is difficult to deny the impact of their drug-induced effects. An exception to this is the case of anxiety. Some psychiatric experts suggest that anxiety is caused by abnormalities of GABA activity, which can be specifically reversed by the action of benzodiazepines on the GABA system. However, even these experts admit that there is little evidence on this point.[1]

Evidence for their usefulness

Short-term studies of benzodiazepines show that they reduce anxiety more than a placebo. However, it is not certain whether this effect persists, since the body adapts to counteract their effects. This is how people become dependent on them. They lose their initial effect because the body's arousal mechanisms are stepped up, but this causes unpleasant withdrawal symptoms when they are stopped. Within psychiatric hospitals, benzodiazepines are commonly used in emergency situations to sedate people who are disturbed or aggressive; a process known as 'rapid tranquillisation'. In these situations the patients often have to be restrained and they are given the drug by force through an intravenous or intramuscular injection. Not surprisingly, given their sedative properties, studies show that benzodiazepines are more effective than a placebo when used in this way. However, evidence about whether they can reduce disturbed behaviour over a long period is lacking.

Dependence

Someone who uses benzodiazepines for more than a few weeks is likely to experience withdrawal symptoms when they stop them. The symptoms include anxiety, agitation, insomnia and muscle stiffness. Since benzodiazepines suppress nervous activity, stopping them increases the activity of the nervous system. Withdrawal can therefore induce unusual and usually unpleasant sensory experiences such as tingling and numbness, electric shock-like feelings and occasionally delusions and hallucinations. Benzodiazepines also suppress the nervous activity that leads to epileptic fits, and so when they are withdrawn, people are at risk of having an epileptic fit. This is a particular concern if someone has been on high doses for a long period. Withdrawal symptoms are more intense after stopping a short-acting drug such as lorazepam or temazepam, because these are expelled from the body more rapidly. Drugs that are eliminated more slowly allow the body time to re-adapt to being without the drug and hence the withdrawal symptoms are less severe.

There are contrasting views on how difficult it is to withdraw from benzodiazepines. Many people claim the withdrawal process is more difficult than coming off heroin. However, some research suggests that for the majority of people withdrawal is not problematic. For example, a study of people who were prescribed benzodiazepines by their general practitioners found that most people did not have great difficulty in getting off them.[2] Withdrawing from higher doses such as those used by drug abusers may be more difficult, and some people experience difficulties withdrawing from lower doses.

Other adverse effects

Like all sedative drugs, benzodiazepines impair people's ability to perform simple physical and mental tasks like driving and mental arithmetic. As with alcohol, people are often unaware of their impairment and rate themselves as functioning better than they are. It is only after they withdraw from medication that they realise how impaired they actually were.[3] Other effects that derive from the ability of benzodiazepines to suppress nervous activity include confusion, slurring of speech and loss of balance. These effects are more likely to occur in elderly people, and when they do, elderly people can have falls and suffer other accidents as a consequence of being oversedated. At very high doses, like other sedative drugs, benzodiazepines suppress the respiratory system and cause death.

A few studies have looked at whether long-term use of benzodiazepines affects the structure of the brain. Two of these studies found a reduction in the amount of brain matter after long-term use of benzodiazepines, similar to findings with neuroleptics.[4,5] However, two other studies found no effects.[6,7]

There has been some concern that benzodiazepines may occasionally lead to disinhibited behaviour and aggression. This mainly seems to occur when high doses are used in people with a prior history of behavioural problems and in people with more vulnerable brains, like children, the elderly and people with learning disability.[8]

The main concerns when using benzodiazepines, however, are the problems of dependence and oversedation.

Considering when to use benzodiazepines

Despite the concerns outlined here, benzodiazepines are probably safer than all the other sorts of drugs commonly used in psychiatry. They do not cause the heart problems associated with neuroleptics that can lead to sudden death. They do not affect weight or metabolism like some of the newer neuroleptics and they do not cause Parkinson's symptoms or tardive dyskinesia. Therefore they might be preferable to neuroleptics for the treatment of acute psychiatric problems such as mania or psychosis, where sedation is likely to be beneficial. One interesting study suggested that the use of a benzodiazepine in people with signs of an impending psychotic relapse could help reduce the risk of going on to have a full-blown relapse.[9] The fact that benzodiazepines do not cause the flattening of emotional reactions and restriction of physical activity that is associated with the neuroleptics means they may not be so unpleasant to take. On the other hand, for the same reason, they may not be so effective in suppressing psychotic symptoms. There needs to be more studies to see how useful benzodiazepines used alone without neuroleptics could be in the treatment of psychosis.

Benzodiazepines can help people to sleep, and so they might be useful in someone who is having trouble sleeping. However, this effect will wear off, and if benzodiazepines are taken for more than a few weeks, withdrawing from them will itself produce sleeping difficulties. It is a similar situation with anxiety. Benzodiazepines may have remarkable effects in reducing anxiety initially, but these effects are likely to decline with time. When the drugs are stopped, anxiety will be induced by the process of withdrawal. For this reason it is recommended that benzodiazepines are not used for more than a month in people with insomnia or anxiety.

Chapter 9
The consequences of a drug-centred approach to understanding psychiatric drugs

Disease- or drug-centred models

The research reviewed in the preceding chapters suggests that there is no basis on which to accept a disease-centred account of psychiatric drug treatments. In other words, there is no convincing evidence that psychiatric disorders or symptoms are caused by a chemical imbalance and no evidence that psychiatric drugs exert their effects by correcting such an imbalance. Instead I have argued that a 'drug-centred' model provides a more compelling account of the nature of psychiatric drugs. According to a drug-centred model, psychiatric drugs are viewed as psychoactive substances whose intoxicating effects suppress or mask the problems that we refer to as psychiatric disorders.

For example, the action of the older neuroleptic or antipsychotic drugs can easily be explained by the fact that they produce a state of mild Parkinson's disease, which slows up mental and physical activity and flattens out emotional reactions. It is obvious how these effects can be interpreted as signs of improvement in someone whose thoughts are dominated by psychotic experiences. There are few comparisons between neuroleptic drugs and other drugs that have a similar impact on thoughts and emotions that could help assess whether neuroleptic drugs act in a drug-centred or disease-centred manner. The only study I am aware of that would qualify is the comparison between opium and chlorpromazine, because of the ability of opium and similar drugs to produce a quality of emotional indifference. This study found that opium was just as good as chlorpromazine in improving the symptoms of an acute psychotic or schizophrenic breakdown. In addition comparisons between neuroleptic drugs and benzodiazepines suggest that more general sedatives may not in fact be inferior.

It is also obvious that someone who is in a certain sort of drugged state is less likely to feel intense emotions such as depression. Again comparative studies do not confirm that antidepressants have a specific action on depression. Instead, almost every sort of psychoactive drug that has been tried in depression has been shown, in one study or another, to have similar effects on symptoms to drugs that are regarded as specific antidepressants. Sedative drugs are clearly likely to reduce the symptoms of mania, since mania is a condition characterised by over-arousal. A child or an adult who is given a small dose of stimulants will become more focused and physically subdued due to a mild increase in their level of arousal. The drug-induced effects associated with psychiatric drugs provide a perfectly adequate explanation for how these drugs impact on the people to whom they are prescribed. There is simply no need to suppose that they reverse a hypothetical chemical imbalance or brain disease.

If you accept this account, the question that will surely come to mind is how can the psychiatric profession and most of society have got it so wrong for so long about the nature of psychiatric drugs? How is it that the disease-centred model of drug action has become so dominant when there is no evidence to support it. The history of psychiatry in the twentieth century suggests that it was adopted because the profession was keen to emulate its colleagues in physical medicine. The psychiatric profession was concerned that it was a Cinderella profession, not as highly regarded or as highly paid as doctors in other areas of medicine. In the mid-twentieth century the profession adopted physical treatments like insulin coma therapy, ECT and frontal lobotomy because they created the appearance that psychiatry was just like the rest of medicine. They allowed the old and terrifying asylums to re-invent themselves as 'mental hospitals' and they allowed psychiatric doctors and nurses to get away from the view that they were glorified gaolers. When the new generation of psychiatric drugs came along in the 1950s they took on the role that was previously occupied by the physical treatments. Drugs became psychiatry's emblematic treatment.

Drug treatment was also useful because in contrast to the dangerous and cumbersome physical treatments such as ECT and insulin coma therapy, drugs could be prescribed to outpatients. This allowed psychiatrists to cultivate larger practices and also helped them to fend off competition from non-medical rivals like social workers, psychologists and psychotherapists.[1]

The pharmaceutical industry is also responsible for promoting the idea that drugs act in a disease-specific way. Drug company material frequently refers to chemical imbalances as the basis of mental disorders and suggests that these can be corrected by drugs. Almost any pharmaceutical company website now carries this sort of message. The drug company Pfizer, for example, described the causes of schizophrenia in the following way on a website for one of its products in 2006: 'imbalances of certain brain chemicals are thought to lead to symptoms of the illness. Medicine plays a key role in balancing these chemicals'.[2]

Eli Lilly, makers of Prozac, recently described how 'a growing amount of evidence supports the view that people with depression have an imbalance of the brain's neurotransmitters, the chemicals that allow nerve cells to communicate with each other. Many scientists believe that an imbalance in serotonin may be an important factor in the development and severity of depression'.[3]

On the website for its new blockbuster neuroleptic drug Zyprexa (olanzapine) Eli Lilly describes how 'antipsychotic medicines are believed to work by balancing the chemicals naturally found in the brain'.[4] The use of the word 'naturally' in this statement suggests that the drug is simply reversing an underlying abnormality, without having any 'unnatural' effects of its own.

In contrast, it is noticeable that drugs are never described in drug-centred terms on pharmaceutical company websites. You never see a description of neuroleptics that tells you they reduce your hallucinations by slowing down all your mental processes. You are not informed that SSRIs may help dull your emotions slightly and make you feel a bit drowsy or that tricyclic antidepressants will make you so sleepy that you will have no time or energy left to feel depressed. Even for drugs that are recommended for the treatment of mania, you are not told that they are useful because they are strongly sedating. We are not even told that stimulants work by increasing arousal. These types of descriptions would make more sense of what drugs can and can't do and form a better basis on which people could decide for themselves whether to use them. But instead people are told again and again that they have a disease or a biological abnormality that drugs can help to reverse. This message is repeated on numerous company websites, despite the fact that it cannot be clearly substantiated with scientific evidence. Information produced by professional bodies and charitable groups also promotes this view and it is reported by the media as if it were established fact. This is how psychiatric knowledge has come to be distorted by commercial interests.

The pharmaceutical industry has promoted the disease-centred model because it is respectable. It allows the industry to push psychiatric drugs onto millions of ordinary people but still appear as a shining angel delivering the sick from their affliction. This is because the disease-centred model makes out that drug treatment must be beneficial because drugs are assumed to reverse or help reverse an underlying abnormality. They help to restore the diseased or malfunctioning body towards a normal level of functioning. In contrast a drug-centred model emphasises that psychiatric drugs are psychoactive substances, not inherently different from the drugs that people take to get high. The idea that millions of people who suffer from depression or anxiety should get intoxicated to deal with their problems would not be an acceptable message. The idea that they have a chemical imbalance that needs correcting is much more marketable.

Western governments have also colluded in the notion that psychiatric drugs are curing diseases. The view that psychiatric conditions are simply medical diseases, and that psychiatric drugs cure or reverse them in the same way that insulin can be said to cure diabetes, is appealing to governments for a number of reasons. It tells a simple story about the nature of psychiatric distress and disturbance, and it presents a simple technical solution in the form of a 'pill for every ill'. This means that governments don't have to grapple with the difficult questions that psychiatric problems raise. For example, governments don't have to resolve the dilemma about how to manage difficult and disturbing behaviour that doesn't fulfil the criteria for the implementation of criminal law. Such behaviour is apparently transformed into a medical problem and hence it is removed from governmental and therefore from democratic jurisdiction.

Deciding when drugs might be beneficial

According to the disease-centred model of drug action, if you become mentally ill you need a drug that counteracts the abnormal biological process that is causing your symptoms. Which drugs counteract which symptoms is supposedly decided by scientific research, principally randomised controlled trials. Therefore you need a doctor or expert of some sort first to tell you what condition you have, in other words to make a diagnosis, and then to tell you what the research says is the correct sort of drug for your particular condition. Of course you can do a lot of this for yourself, such as using checklists of symptoms to diagnose yourself, your friends and relatives and reading reports of the scientific studies on the Internet or in the library. But the point is that this way of thinking depends on the notion that the sufferer has a 'disease', or some sort of biological abnormality, which can only be described properly by scientific research. Finding the right intervention requires a specialist technical knowledge and is therefore properly the realm of professionals.

In contrast, a drug-centred model suggests that it is the subjective experience of taking a drug that determines whether it might be useful or not. It is the way a drug makes you feel, its impact on your bodily functions, on the way you think and your emotional reactions that determine whether it might have beneficial effects for a particular situation. Therefore, it is down to the user of psychiatric drugs to decide whether the effects of a drug are likely to be useful to them in their own unique circumstances.

To make this decision, there are two things that people need to understand. First, people need to have detailed information about the range of drug-induced effects that a particular drug can produce. Second, people need to be clear about the precise nature of the problem for which they are seeking drug treatment. They need to be able to clarify to themselves and to prescribers, in what ways they think drugs might be beneficial.

What sorts of states of intoxication are possible with the main types of drug on offer for different sorts of mental distress? Although it is artificial to distinguish different aspects of the global state drugs produce, the following table summarises some

Table 1: Recognised drug-induced effects

	Euphoria	Sedation	Parkinson's-like effects	Emotional indifference or flattening	Emotional exaggeration	Behavioural disinhibition	Increased arousal	Akathisia, agitation
Older neuroleptics		x	x	x				x
Olanzapine, clozapine		x	x (at higher doses only)	x				x (occasional)
Tricyclic antidepressants		x	?	?				?
SSRIs		x (mild)		?			?	x
Sodium valproate		x		?				
Lithium		x		x				
Stimulants	x	x						
Benzodiazepines	x	x			x	x	x	
Alcohol	x	x			x	x		
Opiates	x	x		x				

of the recognised effects of the psychoactive drugs used in psychiatry. I have done this because it provides a useful starting point for thinking about when and why certain drugs might be useful and, importantly, when they might not be.

Most of the drugs that are commonly used produce sedation. However, the quality of the sedation differs between the different sorts of drugs. Benzodiazepines produce a drowsiness that is associated with feelings of calmness and relaxation, and is experienced as pleasant. In contrast, neuroleptics and tricyclic antidepressants produce an unpleasant feeling of being slow and impaired. Some psychoactive drugs produce effects that are generally experienced as pleasant, and may be sought after by recreational drug users. We say that these drugs cause euphoria. Some psychoactive drugs are commonly disliked, or produce dysphoria (the opposite of euphoria). However, there is great variation in how different individuals respond to different sorts of drugs. Thus although most people dislike the effects of neuroleptics, some people will find them tolerable or even pleasant. Similarly, although being under the influence of benzodiazepines or opiates is generally enjoyed, some people dislike their effects.

Neuroleptic or antipsychotic drugs induce a Parkinson's-like state, with slowing up of mental and physical activity. They also flatten out emotional responses. Opiates also produce a feeling of emotional indifference, or a sort of mental anaesthesia. In contrast, some drugs, such as alcohol and benzodiazepines, exaggerate emotional responses and cause people to act in a disinhibited way. These sorts of drugs commonly make people angry, maudlin and aggressive.

An important point to make here is that the experience of being under the influence of a drug is quite distinct from our normal emotions and experiences. Drugs do not cause genuine happiness, sadness, confidence, pride or envy for example. Some people have talked of drugs like Prozac being lifestyle drugs, or 'smart' drugs, that could make normal people happier, more confident and more successful. But we have no reason to believe that drugs can do anything as sophisticated as this. We have known for a long time that stimulants can enhance performance temporarily, as a consequence of increasing arousal. But this does not make someone more intelligent. As shown in the Table some drugs make you euphoric. However, being euphoric is not the same as being happy. A drug-induced depression, such as occurs with stimulants in children, or with long-term neuroleptics, is different from an ordinary episode of depression in that it is obviously linked to the other suppressing effects of the drug and is not an understandable emotional response to an event in a person's life.

It is also worth pointing out that all psychoactive drugs, because they produce a drug-induced mental state, alter and impair a person's sensitivity to their environment and to the people around them. We can use our knowledge of the effects of alcohol as an example here. When someone is extremely drunk, it is obvious that they are incapable of taking notice or care of anyone or anything, often including themselves. However, the effects of even a small amount of alcohol are often obvious to someone who is sober. People become more self-centred and less aware of other people's needs and emotions than they would normally be. They become bolder, brasher and less discriminating and they are less able to communicate sensitively or to show empathy. Although alcohol produces its own distinctive effects, the feature of reduced sensitivity is common to all states of intoxication produced by mind-altering substances. When the mind is under the influence of a drug, the effects of the drug reduce our normal ability to relate to the world around us.

Of course, when people are severely mentally disordered, their ability to interact appropriately and sensitively is usually impaired. People who are preoccupied with delusional ideas, or people who are in extreme states such as depression or mania, find it difficult to relate to other people normally. In this case a mild level of drug-induced intoxication may improve their ability to interact with people. But if someone takes a psychoactive drug when their mental state is stable, they are likely to be rendered less sensitive to all the things that are taking place around them.

Another consideration is that due to the body's adaptive processes, many drug-induced effects are temporary. For example, drugs that produce euphoria, or give people a buzz, only do so initially. If someone continues to take them, the euphoric effects decline. The user will need to take larger and larger doses to achieve the same 'high' and eventually, if they keep taking the drug they will not get high at all, but simply need to take the drug to avoid getting withdrawal symptoms.

So the range of effects that drugs can produce is limited, and many of the effects are temporary and not sustained. This is the first important piece of information that people should have when considering the use of drugs for psychological disorders. Drugs are blunt instruments. They are unlikely to represent the solution to many people's problems.

The next important thing to clarify when considering using a psychiatric drug is the nature of the problem. Only after a problem is properly understood is it possible to decide if a drug-induced state is likely to be helpful. Drug company propaganda is so widespread that people often approach their doctors nowadays asking for antidepressants or other drugs to treat their 'chemical imbalance'. So it is necessary to work out what the problem actually is. How do people feel exactly, what has precipitated their feelings and how do they think that drug-induced effects can help them? For example, if someone feels sad and lonely after a relationship break-up or bereavement, it is important to explain that there are no drugs that will reverse the underlying feelings. Indeed, many people would argue that the feelings are a necessary part of adapting to and overcoming a major change in life's circumstances. However, there are numerous drugs that will suppress people's emotions by making them feel groggy, sedated and mentally and emotionally flattened, but I suspect this is not what most people are looking for in this situation. On the other hand if someone hasn't slept for a week because they are anxious about something, it might be useful for them to take a drug such as a benzodiazepine, that will temporarily help them to sleep better. A few good nights' sleep might enable them to take steps to tackle the problem that is making them anxious in the first place. However, people need to be aware that the beneficial effects of drugs like benzodiazepines are likely to be short lived. As the body gets used to the drug, its effects will wear off and there are likely to be difficulties in stopping the drug if it is taken for a prolonged period.

Similarly if someone is concerned about a friend or relative, it is important to know what aspects of their behaviour are actually causing concern in order to work out if a drug might be able to influence the situation. If someone with mania is over-aroused, hyperactive and not sleeping, then sedative drugs might be helpful. If someone is repeatedly drunk and abusive due to deep-rooted emotional difficulties, then it is unlikely that taking any sort of drug will prevent this occurring.

Implications for the chemical imbalance theory of psychiatric disorders

In itself, a drug-centred approach to understanding psychiatric drugs does not contradict the idea that psychiatric conditions might be caused by brain abnormalities, or a chemical imbalance. The argument that psychiatric drugs produce drug-induced effects holds, whatever the nature and causes of psychiatric problems. For example, the drug-centred model of drug action does not imply that psychiatric disorders are entirely independent of brain events. Obviously people's behaviour is reflected in the chemistry of their brains. Nor does it imply that there may not be subtle deviations in the brains of some people who require psychiatric care. In fact the drug-centred model is entirely compatible with the view that mental disorders are diseases of the brain, just as diabetes is a disease of the pancreas gland, and cirrhosis is a disease of the liver. All the drug-centred model actually suggests is that the drugs we have at present do not appear to act by reversing a biological defect.

However, the drug-centred model does challenge *current* theories that psychiatric problems are symptoms of an underlying brain disease. This is because the drug-centred model undermines the disease-centred model of drug action; that is, the assumption that psychiatric drugs work by reversing part of an underlying disease process. This disease-centred view of what psychiatric drugs do is held to be the strongest piece of evidence supporting the idea that psychiatric disorders are caused by abnormalities in brain function. The drug-centred model, by suggesting that psychiatric drugs work in an entirely different fashion, means that the action of drugs can no longer be considered to support the view that psychiatric disorders are brain diseases. The action of drugs is important because, as we have seen in discussing the dopamine theory of schizophrenia and the monoamine hypothesis of depression, there is little other evidence that psychiatric symptoms are produced by brain chemical abnormalities. In particular there is no evidence that there are consistent chemical deviations in the brains of people with mental disorders that can be specifically linked to the production of their problems or 'symptoms'.

So, in principle, the drug-centred approach to understanding the nature of psychiatric drugs is compatible with biological *or* social explanations of the nature and origins of psychiatric conditions. However, the drug-centred model undermines the view that psychiatric disorders are equivalent to brain diseases because the assumption that psychiatric drugs act in a disease-centred manner, which the drug-centred model challenges, has always been one of the strongest arguments put forward to support this view.

Chapter 10
Withdrawing from psychiatric drugs

According to the principles set out in this book, many people are currently prescribed psychiatric drugs that give them no benefit and that may cause them harm, especially over the long term. Therefore some people might want to consider stopping, or at least reducing, their drug treatment. This process can be difficult for a variety of reasons and the difficulties may unfortunately lead many people to abandon the attempt to give up their drugs. Although there are recognised adverse effects when someone stops psychiatric medication that they have taken for a long time, the difficulties are often compounded because they are not recognised as withdrawal effects. Instead they are usually interpreted as the re-emergence of the underlying problem and taken as confirmation of the need for life-long treatment. If withdrawal-related effects are recognised for what they are, there are a number of ways to manage them without necessarily restarting long-term medication.

Before describing the various withdrawal-related problems it is also worth pointing out that they do not occur in all people, and some people who do experience withdrawal effects do not find them problematic. Some people will be able to stop their drug treatment quite easily. This especially applies to people who have been taking drug treatment for shorter periods. In general the longer you have been taking something the harder it may be to withdraw. However, even in this situation not everyone experiences problems.

The following problems are known to occur after stopping drug treatment:

1. *Withdrawal symptoms*

We now know that all psychoactive drugs produce withdrawal or discontinuation syndromes that include physical and psychological symptoms. Withdrawal symptoms are caused by the body's response to the withdrawal of a drug it had got used to. When someone takes a drug on a long-term basis the body makes adaptations to try and counter the effects of the drug. For example, people taking dopamine receptor-blocking drugs like the neuroleptics will manufacture more dopamine receptors in their brains, and those that exist will change and become more sensitive to dopamine. This is the body's way of trying to increase the activity of dopamine despite the presence of a chemical that tends to reduce its activity. When the drug is stopped, these extra dopamine receptors will still be present, and may increase the activity of dopamine above normal levels until they reduce back down to normal numbers. Usually the body's adaptations disappear gradually when the drug is no longer present and the symptoms subside. However, we know very little about the body's response to long-term drug treatment and how the body reacts to the withdrawal of such treatment. It is possible that the adaptations sometimes persist. For example, we know that the abnormal movements of tardive dyskinesia often get worse when neuroleptic drugs are reduced or stopped. This is likely to be mediated by the increased numbers and activity of dopamine receptors. Sometimes the movements improve with time as the body readjusts to the fact the drug has been stopped. However, sometimes they are permanent, implying that the adaptation of the body's dopamine system to the presence of neuroleptics can be irreversible.

Most psychiatric drugs affect a range of different brain chemicals or neurotransmitters, and withdrawal effects can reflect the drug's impact on any of these chemical systems. Withdrawal symptoms themselves may be mild and annoying, they may be unpleasant and sometimes they are unbearable. In addition withdrawal from sedative drugs often causes agitation and insomnia, which can easily be mistaken for early signs of relapse. When drugs have been taken for a long time, such as several years, it is possible that the body will take a considerable time to readjust and withdrawal symptoms may go on for some time.

2. *Withdrawal-related psychosis*

There is evidence from case reports and small studies that stopping neuroleptic or antipsychotic drugs can sometimes provoke psychotic symptoms.[1] This has been reported in some people who had no previous psychiatric history and were placed on neuroleptic-type drugs for physical problems. The symptoms appear to be caused directly by the drug withdrawal. In other words they are part of the withdrawal state. Some authors refer to this condition as 'supersensitivity psychosis'. This term is based on the idea that the symptoms are caused by the dopamine receptors becoming supersensitive to dopamine, due to the presence of dopamine-blocking drugs. However, this has never been proven, and it is likely that other mechanisms are also involved.

The evidence suggests it is most likely to occur after withdrawal of clozapine. Clozapine is rapidly eliminated from the body compared with other neuroleptic drugs and therefore stopping clozapine is likely to result in a more severe withdrawal syndrome. Since clozapine has weaker effects on dopamine receptors than other neuroleptics, this would suggest that a psychotic withdrawal reaction is not entirely due to dopamine system dysfunction.

This type of reaction is worrying not just for its own sake, but because when it occurs in people who have had a previous episode of psychosis, it is likely to be interpreted as the re-emergence of the underlying disorder. In this case everyone will believe that the withdrawal process has failed. The individual will almost certainly be told that they must restart medication and no further attempts will be made to withdraw it.

3. *Relapse precipitated by withdrawal*

Some research suggests that stopping certain psychiatric drugs can provoke a relapse of the underlying psychiatric condition. In other words someone who stops long-term psychiatric drug treatment may be more likely to have a relapse than they would have been if they had never started it. Alternatively it could be viewed that stopping long-term treatment brings forward a relapse that might otherwise have occurred later. We are not sure how this happens, but it may be because an intense withdrawal reaction is a stressful experience and we know that stressful events may precipitate an episode of mental illness.

This effect has been shown most clearly in the case of lithium. People with manic depression who stop lithium are more likely to have a relapse, especially a manic one, than they were before they started it.[2] There is also evidence that people with schizophrenia or psychotic disorders who take neuroleptics on a long-term basis may have an increased risk of relapse after stopping them.[3] Most studies suggest that slow or gradual reduction reduces the risk of relapse, maybe because the experience of withdrawal is less stressful and the body has time to re-adapt to the absence of the drug.

Once again, the occurrence of a relapse after withdrawal or reduction of a drug is usually interpreted as confirming the need for ongoing treatment. Therefore medication is usually restarted if it has been stopped, or increased back to its original level if it has been reduced. Further attempts to reduce or stop medication will almost certainly be discouraged.

4. *Psychological dependence*

Finally, people may become psychologically dependent on taking medication and may become anxious if they know or suspect that they have been withdrawn from it. Again, the anxiety may be mistaken for a relapse of the original condition, or it may even precipitate a relapse.

Withdrawing from psychiatric drugs has some similarities with giving up recreational drugs. For example, people may become dependent on psychiatric drugs in both physical and psychological senses, as they do with drugs of abuse. The only real difference is that drugs of abuse have pleasant effects. They make people high, and so people crave the drug when they stop it. In contrast, people do not usually crave the effects of drugs such as neuroleptics. However, many people who have taken psychiatric drugs for years on end will find it difficult to adjust to being in an undrugged state. In the same way that alcoholics and drug addicts often have to go through 'rehab' programmes to learn to live life without drugs, so long-term users of psychiatric medication cannot necessarily adjust overnight. For example, they will have to learn or relearn how to deal with normal emotional reactions after years of having them suppressed by drugs. They will have to learn how to deal with difficult social situations without embarrassment, anger or other emotional reactions that they may not have experienced for many years. After years of taking sedatives that make people sleep a lot of the time, and feel so groggy the rest of the time that they don't wish to do anything, people have to learn how to fill their time again. People have to find ways of occupying their minds and their bodies so that they don't get bored, lonely or frustrated, feelings that may have been suppressed by drug treatment.

In the current climate that puts so much emphasis on the benefits of prescribed drugs, it takes a lot of courage to decide to come off them. Often there is little help for people who decide to do so. However, some local support groups have started up in the United Kingdom, and recently one of these has developed a website which provides information for people wishing to reduce or stop their psychiatric medication, and helps put people in touch with others who are trying to do this, or who have successfully done so (www.comingoff.com). Another service user group based in the United States, the Icarus Project, has developed a detailed guideline about coming off medication, which is available from their website (details of these and other sources of support are listed in the Appendix).

There is no right or wrong way to come off psychiatric medication in most cases. It is down to each individual to decide what suits them best. However, there are a few cases where sudden withdrawal can be dangerous, like withdrawal from high-dose benzodiazepines, alcohol or barbiturates. Rapid withdrawal of high-dose benzodiazepines, alcohol and barbiturates can cause epileptic fits and a severe withdrawal reaction that can be life threatening in itself. In these circumstances it is very important that withdrawal is carried out slowly and carefully with medical supervision. Substitution of short-acting drugs with long-acting drugs is important in the case of benzodiazepine withdrawal, so temazepam and lorazepam are converted to diazepam (Valium) or chlordiazepoxide (Librium). Long-acting benzodiazepines, reduced gradually, are also used to reduce the intensity of alcohol withdrawal symptoms.

Slow or gradual withdrawal is also likely to reduce the risk of developing a withdrawal-related psychotic reaction after stopping neuroleptic drugs due to the lower intensity of the body's reaction after slow withdrawal. Therefore it is advisable that everyone who has been taking neuroleptics for a long period should reduce them gradually. This is especially important for neuroleptics with short half-lives (see below), or rapid elimination from the body, such as clozapine, sulpiride and amisulpiride. Similarly, it seems likely that slow withdrawal will reduce the likelihood of having a relapse precipitated by the withdrawal process. Since this has been shown to occur most consistently after lithium withdrawal, I would advise everyone who wants to come off lithium to reduce it as gradually as possible.

In general, if you stop taking something suddenly, the withdrawal symptoms will be more intense, but they will last for a shorter period. If you reduce a drug gradually the withdrawal symptoms will be less intense, and may be so mild that you will not notice them at all. Different drugs differ in their ability to cause withdrawal symptoms. 'Short-acting' drugs that act quickly and are rapidly eliminated from the body cause more intense withdrawal symptoms than 'long-acting' drugs that stay around in the body for longer. The rate of elimination of a drug is measured in what is called its 'half-life'. A half-life means the time it takes for the concentration in the body to decline by half. Drugs with a short half-life are eliminated rapidly, while drugs with a long half-life remain in the body for longer. Heroin, for example, has a short half-life and causes more symptoms after stopping than methadone, which has a long half-life. This is the principle behind the practice of prescribing methadone to heroin addicts to help them withdraw. Fluoxetine (Prozac) is another example of a drug with a long half-life. It is eliminated from the body slowly over a period of weeks. Therefore you can stop it suddenly, and its effects will naturally wear off gradually. It is the same with the depot preparations of neuroleptic drugs, which are given by an intramuscular injection every few weeks. Depot preparations are designed to deliver drugs slowly over a long period and therefore the dose of the drug in the body declines gradually after each injection. In contrast, drugs such as lorazepam, paroxetine and clozapine are eliminated rapidly from the body – they have short half-lives. That is why you have to take repeated doses of them every day to get an even amount of the drug in the body over a daily period. These drugs cause more intense withdrawal symptoms when stopped.

Therefore if you are considering withdrawing from a prescribed medication it is important to know what are called the 'pharmacodynamic' properties of the drug you are taking. This means knowing about the rate of elimination of a drug; in other words knowing its half-life. A psychiatric pharmacist will probably be the best person to give you this information and each mental health trust has a pharmacy department. If you are taking a drug with a short half-life you know you will experience more intense withdrawal symptoms if you stop it suddenly, and you might wish to transfer to something longer acting, with a longer half-life. However, withdrawing from a long-acting preparation may cause milder but protracted withdrawal symptoms that go on for months. So some people may decide it is better to get the withdrawal process over and done with, and prefer to simply stop the short-acting preparation. It is an individual decision, and much depends on how each individual copes with the discomfort and disruption caused by withdrawal. Some people throw their tablets away and stop taking them overnight and it works. Other people find the withdrawal symptoms excruciating, and have to reduce their dose of medication very gradually over a period of months or even years. The most important thing is to be prepared. It may be possible to endure severe withdrawal symptoms as long as you know they will be short-lived. If you don't know what the symptoms are caused by or how long they will last, the experience is more likely to be unbearable.

If someone who tries to stop their medication gets into difficulties, it does not necessarily mean that the process of withdrawal must be abandoned. If people are aware that various problems may arise from the withdrawal process itself, and are likely to improve with time, it may be possible to manage the situation without simply resuming the previous levels of drug treatment. For example, someone who experiences severe withdrawal symptoms, or a withdrawal-related psychosis, could have a temporary increase in their neuroleptic medication, followed by a more gradual withdrawal schedule, once they had stabilised. For some people, extra support over the period of withdrawal and access to emergency care may tide them over difficult periods. Intensive psychotherapy may help people to cope with withdrawal symptoms, reduce stress levels and enable people to identify alternative coping mechanisms.

People who decide to come off their medication, however they decide to do it, should have adequate information on which to base their decision, an opportunity to talk through the pros and cons of different options, and the availability of extra support through the withdrawal period. Remember that although most doctors and other professional staff will not recommend stopping psychiatric medication, they cannot force people to take it unless they are subject to the Mental Health Act. Unless you are in this situation, it is down to you whether you take psychiatric medication or not. If you make a thoughtful and considered decision to try and stop or reduce your drug treatment, your mental health team should support you through this process. However, if professional staff undermine you by continually telling you that coming off medication will fail, you may need to seek help from other service users and organisations with more positive attitudes to stopping medication.

Chapter 11
Final thoughts

Based on the analysis presented in this book, there is a
minimum set of questions that people should ask if they are
considering starting a psychiatric drug, or if they are already
taking one. Because research on psychiatric drugs has been so
preoccupied with the disease-centred model of drug action,
most of the questions do not have answers. However, it is not
until we start asking the right questions that the research
community will start to conduct research that can provide the
answers.

1. The first question to ask about a psychiatric drug that a
doctor proposes to prescribe is what sort of drug-induced
state does the drug produce? Is the drug predominantly
sedative or stimulant? What are the drug's effects on
thought processes, emotions and behaviour in normal
people?

2. We need to ask what happens when the drug is used
continuously for long periods? Do the acute effects persist
or are they lost due to the body's adaptations? What other
effects emerge? Do you need to keep increasing the dose to
maintain the initial effect?

3. We should demand evidence about the effects of long-
term use on the structure and function of the brain and
other parts of the body.

4. We need information about what physical and mental symptoms are produced when the drug is stopped.

5. People should ask whether the drug is short- or long-acting and how long is its half-life. In other words how long does it stay around in the body after a single dose?

6. Everyone who considers using a psychiatric drug should ask what is known about the chances of recovering without drug treatment.

7. People should know what sort of evidence exists that using a drug in their particular situation will help them improve.

8. If long-term treatment has been started or is being considered, people should ask about the evidence for the value of long-term treatment.

9. People should be informed about the deficiencies of that evidence. Have studies used withdrawal designs for example, or ignored likely unblinding effects?

10. Everyone should be given information about what alternatives are available to using drugs.

11. People should ask if the mental health services will support them if they choose not to use drugs, or to use them briefly and then stop them, even if this is not what is recommended.

Unfortunately people have to make judgements about whether to take drugs and how long to continue them for on the basis of totally inadequate information. In this situation the severity of the problem and whether any alternative avenues are available are likely to be important considerations. Counselling and short-term psychotherapy should now be available to people in the United Kingdom with mental distress, through their general practitioners. This is a welcome alternative to the ubiquitous prescribing of antidepressants. Unfortunately there are few choices for people with severe psychiatric problems. Although research studies conducted in Finland and the United States showed that 30–40% of people with a first episode of a psychotic disorder can be successfully treated without using any neuroleptic medication, in general, it is extremely difficult to avoid being medicated for a psychotic condition nowadays. And, once medicated, it is difficult to stop the medication, for all the reasons described in the preceding chapter. Therefore people with a severe psychiatric disorder like psychosis inevitably end up taking neuroleptic drugs for years on end, even though this may be avoidable for at least some of them.

Conclusions

In this book I have argued that the current assumptions about how psychiatric drugs work and what they do are erroneous. I have suggested that psychiatric drugs do not reverse an underlying biological abnormality, as suggested by the orthodox 'disease-centred' view of what they do; they in fact create one. The drugs used in psychiatry are psychoactive chemicals that cause an altered drug-induced state, a state of intoxication, in other words. Although people have assumed that the disease-centred model is true for over half a century now, there is no evidence to support it. When we acknowledge that psychiatric drugs are psychoactive drugs, it is obvious that they will exert effects that will alter, suppress or obscure the manifestations of psychological and emotional problems. These effects may easily be mistaken for an improvement in the underlying condition if that is all that people are looking for.

A 'drug-centred' model views drugs as producing abnormal states that may occasionally be useful for people with psychiatric problems. This model emphasises that drugs produce drug-induced effects, and that these effects are not the same as normal experiences. Drugs do not simply reproduce ordinary emotional states. They produce characteristic altered states, which vary according to the pharmacological properties of the drug concerned. Drugs are not a sophisticated way of restoring or enhancing normal functioning. They are just drugs. They can make you fast or slow, euphoric or dysphoric. They can produce some curious and usually unpleasant experiences and sensations. But they do not make a troubled person happy or a disturbed person normal. They can be useful because, when someone is very distressed, it may be preferable to be in a drug-induced state. As Peter Breggin points out, 'biopsychiatric treatments are deemed effective when the physician and/or the patient prefer a state of diminished brain function with its narrowed range of mental capacity or emotional expression'.[1]

The drug-centred model suggests that the relationship between the patient and the prescriber should be different. Service users and their friends, family and carers should no longer simply accept that the doctor makes a diagnosis and tells them what treatment is deemed appropriate for it. They should ask and debate with their doctor about what sort of drug-induced effects might be useful in their particular situation. They should explore by themselves and with others what the benefits of a drug-induced state would be and what negative consequences are likely to flow from that state. They should also have the opportunity to consider the use of alternatives to drug treatment.

People who are already on drug treatment might want to reflect on what drug-induced effects they are experiencing, and how these effects might be impacting on their lives. They will want to balance any positive effects they feel they obtain against the negative or unpleasant effects and the evidence for long-term harm. People who want to stop their drug treatment, either because they are stable, or because they feel it has not helped, will need information about the nature of the drug they are on before they can decide the best method for coming off it. So the drug-centred model makes the patient the expert in their own drug treatment. It is up to them to decide whether they find certain effects useful or not. However, in order to do this, patients and professionals have to understand the limitations of what drug treatment can achieve.

Thus the drug-centred approach demands that everyone from consumers to pharmaceutical researchers become more informed about the nature of the drugs that are prescribed to people with psychiatric problems. For this to be possible, there needs to be more research into the characteristic effects of different drugs as well as the long-term consequences of taking them. The drug-centred model also highlights how taking psychiatric drugs is always a delicate balancing act between benefits and harm. The useful effects that drugs have are part and parcel of a drug-induced state, a state of intoxication, that is not the same as the ordinary state of the body. Taking psychoactive drugs is likely to impair and suppress aspects of our mental and emotional life. The question is whether that impairment is preferable to the psychiatric distress that is being experienced. Sometimes the distress will be so severe that a level of drug-induced suppression will be greeted with welcome relief. In other situations people may find the effects of the drugs so unpleasant that they prefer to be in a state of mental turmoil.

Although most people are advised to take psychiatric drugs for long periods after their psychiatric problems have subsided, the evidence on which these recommendations is based is seriously flawed because of the neglect of the impact of withdrawal effects on studies of long-term treatment. We know that long-term use of certain drugs, especially neuroleptics, produces harmful and sometimes dangerous effects, but we are not certain that it is beneficial from the point of view of improving the course of the psychiatric condition. Therefore people who refuse long-term treatment, or who decide to stop it are not behaving irrationally, as often assumed, but are making a perfectly legitimate and well-founded decision. There should be more support available for people who want to try and cope without drug treatment.

A drug-centred approach to psychiatric drugs emphasises that their effects are crude and their ability to improve the lives of people who experience psychiatric problems is limited. They are widely over-prescribed at present, even according to conventional psychiatric standards. Hopefully setting out an alternative way of understanding their effects, as I have attempted in this book, will enable people to make a more realistic appraisal of the likely risks ands benefits involved in using psychiatric drugs.

Endnotes

Chapter 1

1. Moncrieff, J (1999) An investigation into the precedents of modern drug treatment in psychiatry. *Hist Psychiatry 10*(40 Pt 4), 475–90.

2. Braslow, J (1997) *Mental Ills and Bodily Cures*. Berkely, CA: University of California Press.

3. Szasz, T (1970) *Ideology and Insanity: Essays on the psychiatric dehumanization of man.* New York: Anchor Books.

4. Moncrieff, J (2008) The creation of the concept of the antidepressant: An historical analysis. *Social Science and Medicine 66*(11), 2346–55.

5. Healy, D (2004) Shaping the intimate: Influences on the experience of everyday nerves. *Soc.Stud.Sci. 34*(2), 219–45.

6. Heres, S, Davis, J, Maino, K, Jetzinger, E, Kissling, W & Leucht, S (2006) Why olanzapine beats risperidone, risperidone beats quetiapine, and quetiapine beats olanzapine: An exploratory analysis of head-to-head comparison studies of second-generation antipsychotics. *Am.J.Psychiatry 163*(2), 185–94.

Chapter 2

1. Moncrieff, J (1999) An investigation into the precedents of modern drug treatment in psychiatry. *Hist Psychiatry 10*(40 Pt 4), 475–90.

2. Moncrieff, J & Cohen, D (2006) Do antidepressants cure or create abnormal brain states? *PLoS.Med. 3*(7), e240.

3. Lacasse, JR & Leo, J (2005) Serotonin and depression: A disconnect between the advertisements and the scientific literature. *PLoS.Med. 2*(12), e392.

4. For more information, see Moncrieff J (2009) A critique of the dopamine hypothesis of schizophrenia and psychosis. *Harv.Rev.Psychiatry*.

5. Deniker, P (1960) Experimental neurological syndromes and the new drug therapies in psychiatry. *Compr.Psychiatry 1*, 92–102.

6. Moncrieff, J (2008) *The Myth of the Chemical Cure: A critique of psychiatric drug treatment.* Basingstoke: Palgrave Macmillan.

7. Moncrieff, J & Cohen, D (2005) Rethinking models of psychotropic drug action. *Psychother.Psychosom. 74*(3), 145–53.

8. See n. 6.

9. See n. 7.

Chapter 3

1. Melander, H, Ahlqvist-Rastad, J, Meijer, G & Beermann, B (2003) Evidence b(i)ased medicine – Selective reporting from studies sponsored by pharmaceutical industry: Review of studies in new drug applications. *BMJ 326*(7400), 1171–3.

2. Ibid.

3. Jureidini, JN, McHenry, LB & Mansfield, PR (2008) Clinical trials and drug promotion: Selective reporting of study 329. *International Journal of Risk and Safety in Medicine 20*(1-2), 73–81.

4. Lasagna, L, Masteller, F, von Flesinger, JM & Beecher, HK (1954) A study of the placebo response. *American Journal of Medicine 16*, 770–9.

5. Fisher, S & Greenberg, RP (1993) How sound is the double-blind design for evaluating psychotropic drugs? *J.Nerv.Ment.Dis. 181*(6), 345–50.

6. Moncrieff, J (2006) Why is it so difficult to stop psychiatric drug treatment? It may be nothing to do with the original problem. *Med.Hypotheses 67*(3), 517–23.

7. Raskin, A, Schulterbrandt, JG, Reatig, N & McKeon, JJ (1970) Differential response to chlorpromazine, imipramine, and placebo. A study of subgroups of hospitalized depressed patients. *Arch.Gen.Psychiatry 23*(2), 164–73.

8. Kirsch, I & Moncrieff, J (2007) Clinical trials and the response rate illusion. *Contemp.Clin.Trials 28*, 348–51.

9. Cohen, D & Jacobs, D (2007) Randomized controlled trials of antidepressants: Clinically and scientifically irrelevant. Debates in *Neuroscience 1*, 44–54.

Chapter 4

1. Belmaker, RH & Wald, D (1977) Haloperidol in normals. *Br.J.Psychiatry 131*, 222–3.

2. Healy, D & Farquhar, G (1998) Immediate effects of droperidol. *Hum.Psychopharmacol. 13*, 113–20.

3. Breggin, PR (1993) *Toxic Psychiatry*. London: Fontana.

4. Ramaekers, JG, Louwerens, JW, Muntjewerff, ND, Milius, H, de Bie, A, Rosenzweig, P et al (1999) Psychomotor, cognitive, extrapyramidal, and affective functions of healthy volunteers during treatment with an atypical (amisulpride) and a classic (haloperidol) antipsychotic. *J.Clin.Psychopharmacol. 19*(3), 209–21.

5. McClelland, GR, Cooper, SM & Pilgrim, AJ (1990) A comparison of the central nervous system effects of haloperidol, chlorpromazine and sulpiride in normal volunteers. *Br.J.Clin.Pharmacol. 30*(6), 795–803.

6. Gemperle, AY, McAllister, KH & Olpe, HR (2003) Differential effects of iloperidone, clozapine, and haloperidol on working memory of rats in the delayed non-matching-to-position paradigm. *Psychopharmacology (Berl) 169*(3-4), 354–64.

7. Moncrieff, J, Cohen, D & Mason, JP (in press) The subjective experience of taking antipsychotic medication: A content analysis of internet data. *Acta Psychiatr.Scand.*

8. Seidman, LJ, Pepple, JR, Faraone, SV, Kremen, WS, Green, AI, Brown, WA & Tsuang, MT (1993) Neuropsychological performance in chronic schizophrenia in response to neuroleptic dose reduction. *Biol.Psychiatry 33*(8-9), 575–84.

9. Abse, DW, Dahlstrom, WG &Tolley, AG (1960) Evaluation of tranquilizing drugs in the management of acute mental disturbance. *Am.J.Psychiatry* 116, 973–80.

10. Wolkowitz, OM & Pickar, D (1991) Benzodiazepines in the treatment of schizophrenia: A review and reappraisal. *Am.J.Psychiatry 148*(6), 714–26.

11. Casey, JF, Lasky, JJ, Klett, CJ & Hollister, LE (1960) Treatment of schizophrenic reactions with phenothiazine derivatives. A comparative study of chlorpromazine, triflupromazine, mepazine, prochlorperazine, perphenazine, and phenobarbital. *Am.J.Psychiatry* 117, 97–105.

12. Casey, JF, Bennett, IF, Lindley, CJ, Hollister, LE, Gordon, MH & Springer, NN (1960) Drug therapy in schizophrenia. A controlled study of the relative effectiveness of chlorpromazine, promazine, phenobarbital, and placebo. *Arch.Gen.Psychiatry 2*, 210–20.

13. Bola, JR & Mosher, LR (2003) Treatment of acute psychosis without neuroleptics: Two-year outcomes from the Soteria project. *J.Nerv.Ment.Dis. 191*(4), 219–29.

14. Lehtinen, V, Aaltonen, J, Koffert, T, Rakkolainen, V & Syvalahti, E (2000) Two-year outcome in first-episode psychosis treated according to an integrated model. Is immediate neuroleptisation always needed? *Eur.Psychiatry 15*(5), 312–20.

15. Moncrieff, J (2003) Clozapine v. conventional antipsychotic drugs for treatment-resistant schizophrenia: A re-examination. *Br.J.Psychiatry 183*, 161–6.

16. Viguera, AC, Baldessarini, RJ, Hegarty, JD, van Kammen, DP & Tohen, M (1997) Clinical risk following abrupt and gradual withdrawal of maintenance neuroleptic treatment. *Arch.Gen.Psychiatry 54*(1), 49–55.

17. Samaha, AN, Seeman, P, Stewart, J, Rajabi, H & Kapur, S (2007) 'Breakthrough' dopamine supersensitivity during ongoing antipsychotic treatment leads to treatment failure over time. *J.Neurosci. 27*(11), 2979–86.

18. Olfson, M, Blanco, C, Liu, L, Moreno, C & Laje, G (2006) National trends in the outpatient treatment of children and adolescents with antipsychotic drugs. *Arch.Gen.Psychiatry 63*(6), 679–85.

19. Wonodi, I, Reeves, G, Carmichael, D, Verovsky, I, Avila, MT, Elliott, A et al (2007) Tardive dyskinesia in children treated with atypical antipsychotic medications. *Movement Disorder Society 22*(12), 1777–82

20. Waddington, JL & Youssef, HA (1996) Cognitive dysfunction in chronic schizophrenia followed prospectively over 10 years and its longitudinal relationship to the emergence of tardive dyskinesia. *Psychol.Med. 26*(4), 681–8.

21. Breggin, PR (1990) Brain damage, dementia and persistent cognitive dysfunction associated with neuroleptic drugs. Evidence, etiology,

implications. *Journal of Mind and Behaviour 11*, 425–64.

22. Jeste, DV, Caligiuri, MP, Paulsen, JS, Heaton, RK, Lacro, JP, Harris, MJ et al (1995) Risk of tardive dyskinesia in older patients. A prospective longitudinal study of 266 outpatients. *Arch.Gen.Psychiatry 52*(9), 756–65.

23. Lieberman, JA, Tollefson, GD, Charles, C, Zipursky, R, Sharma, T, Kahn, RS et al (2005) Antipsychotic drug effects on brain morphology in first-episode psychosis. *Arch. Gen. Psychiatry 62*(4), 361–70.

24. Dazzan, P, Morgan, KD, Orr, K, Hutchinson, G, Chitnis, X, Suckling, J et al (2005) Different effects of typical and atypical antipsychotics on grey matter in first episode psychosis: The AESOP study. *Neuropsychopharmacology 30*(4), 765–74.

25. Joukamaa, M, Heliovaara, M, Knekt, P, Aromaa, A, Raitasalo, R & Lehtinen, V (2006) Schizophrenia, neuroleptic medication and mortality. *Br.J.Psychiatry 188*, 122–7.

26. Davis, JM & Chen, N (2004) Dose response and dose equivalence of antipsychotics. *J.Clin.Psychopharmacol. 24*(2), 192–208.

27. Healthcare Commission (2007) *Talking about Medicines: The management of medicines in Trusts providing mental health services*. London: Commission for Healthcare, Audit and Inspection.

Chapter 5

1. National Institute for Health and Clinical Excellence (2004) *Depression: Management of depression in primary and secondary care. Clinical practice guideline Number 23*. London: National Institute for Health and Clinical Excellence.

2. Stagnitti, M (2005) *Antidepressant Use in the US Civilian Non Institutionalized Population, 2002. Statistical Brief #77*. Rockville, MD: Medical Expenditure Panel, Agency for Healthcare Research and Quality.

3. Heydorn, W, Frazer, A & Mendels, J (1980) Do tricyclic antidepressants enhance adrenergic transmission? An update. *Am.J.Psychiatry 137*(1), 113–14.

4. Schildkraut, JJ, Winokur, A & Applegate, CW (1970) Norepinephrine turnover and metabolism in rat brain after long-term administration of imipramine. *Science 168*(933), 867–9.

5. Schultz, J (1976) Psychoactive drug effects on a system which generates cyclic AMP in brain. *Nature 261*(5559), 417–18.

6. Vetulani, J & Sulser, F (1975) Action of various antidepressant treatments reduces reactivity of noradrenergic cyclic AMP-generating system in limbic forebrain. *Nature 257*(5526), 495–6.

7. Delini-Stula, A & Vassout, A (1979) Modulation of dopamine-mediated behavioural responses by antidepressants: Effects of single and repeated treatment. *Eur.J.Pharmacol. 58*(4), 443–51.

8. Dumont, GJ, de Visser, SJ, Cohen, AF & van Gerven, JM (2005) Biomarkers for the effects of selective serotonin reuptake inhibitors (SSRIs) in healthy subjects. *Br.J.Clin.Pharmacol. 59*(5), 495–510.

9. Herrmann, WM & McDonald, RJ (1978) A multidimensional test approach for the description of the CNS activity of drugs in human pharmacology. *Pharmakopsychiatr.Neuropsychopharmakol. 11*(6), 247–65.

10. See n. 8.

11. Beasley, CM Jr, Sayler, ME, Bosomworth, JC & Wernicke, JF (1991) High-dose fluoxetine: Efficacy and activating-sedating effects in agitated and retarded depression. *Journal of Clinical Psychopharmacology 11*, 166–74.

12. Healy, D, Herxheimer, A & Menkes, DB (2006) Antidepressants and violence: Problems at the interface of medicine and law. *PLoS.Med. 3*(9), e372.

13. Taylor, D, Paton, C & Kerwin, R (2005) *The Maudsley 2005–2006 Prescribing Guidelines*. London: Taylor & Francis.

14. Kirsch, I, Moore, TJ, Scoboria, A & Nicholls, SS (2002) The emperor's new drugs: An analysis of antidepressant medication data submitted to the US Food and Drug Administration. *Prevention and Treatment, 5*, article 23.

15. See n. 1.

16. Joyce, PR & Paykel, ES (1989) Predictors of drug response in depression. *Arch.Gen.Psychiatry 46*(1), 89–99.

17. See n. 1.

18. Moncrieff, J (2003) A comparison of antidepressant trials using active and inert placebos. *Int.J.Methods Psychiatr.Res. 12*(3), 117–27.

19. Khan, A, Leventhal, RM, Khan, SR & Brown, WA (2002) Severity of depression and response to antidepressants and placebo: An analysis of the Food and Drug Administration database. *J.Clin.Psychopharmacol. 22*(1), 40–5.

20. Angst, J, Scheidegger, P & Stabl, M (1993) Efficacy of moclobemide in different patient groups. Results of new subscales of the Hamilton Depression Rating Scale. *Clin.Neuropharmacol. 16* Suppl 2, S55–S62.

21. Kirsch, I, Deacon, BJ, Huedo-Medina, TB, Scoboria, A, Moore, TJ et al (2008) Initial severity and antidepressant benefits: A meta-analysis of data submitted to the Food and Drug Administration. *PLoS Med 5*(2), e45.

22. See n. 13.

23. Teicher, MH, Glod, C & Cole, JO (1990) Emergence of intense suicidal preoccupation during fluoxetine treatment. *Am.J.Psychiatry 147*(2), 207–10.

24. Dubicka, B, Hadley, S & Roberts, C (2006) Suicidal behaviour in youths with depression treated with new-generation antidepressants: Meta-analysis. *Br.J.Psychiatry 189*, 393–8.

25. Olfson, M, Marcus, SC & Shaffer, D (2006) Antidepressant drug therapy and suicide in severely depressed children and adults: A case-control study.

Arch.Gen.Psychiatry 63(8), 865–72.

26. Whittington, CJ, Kendall, T, Fonagy, P, Cottrell, D, Cotgrove, A & Boddington, E (2004) Selective serotonin reuptake inhibitors in childhood depression: Systematic review of published versus unpublished data. *Lancet 363*(9418), 1341–5.

27. Wohlfarth, TD, van Zwieten, BJ, Lekkerkerker, FJ, Gispen-de Wied, CC, Ruis, JR, Elferink, AJ & Storosum, JG (2006) Antidepressants use in children and adolescents and the risk of suicide. *Eur.Neuropsychopharmacol. 16*(2), 79–83.

28. Fergusson, D, Doucette, S, Glass, KC, Shapiro, S, Healy, D, Hebert, P & Hutton, B (2005) Association between suicide attempts and selective serotonin reuptake inhibitors: Systematic review of randomised controlled trials. *BMJ 330*(7488), 396.

29. Gunnell, D, Saperia, J & Ashby, D (2005) Selective serotonin reuptake inhibitors (SSRIs) and suicide in adults: Meta-analysis of drug company data from placebo controlled, randomised controlled trials submitted to the MHRA's safety review. *BMJ 330*(7488), 385.

30. Beasley, CM Jr, Dornseif, BE, Bosomworth, JC, Sayler, ME, Rampey AH Jr, Heiligenstein, JH et al (1991) Fluoxetine and suicide: A meta-analysis of controlled trials of treatment for depression. *BMJ 303*(6804), 685–92.

31. Khan, A, Khan, S, Kolts, R & Brown, WA (2003) Suicide rates in clinical trials of SSRIs, other antidepressants, and placebo: Analysis of FDA reports. *Am.J.Psychiatry 160*(4), 790–2.

32. See n. 28.

33. Martinez, C, Rietbrock, S, Wise, L, Ashby, D, Chick, J, Moseley et al (2005) Antidepressant treatment and the risk of fatal and non-fatal self harm in first episode depression: Nested case-control study. *BMJ 330*(7488), 389.

34. See n. 12.

35. Breggin, PR (1997) *Brain Disabling Treatments in Psychiatry: Drugs, electroshock and the role of the FDA.* New York: Springer Publishing Company.

36. Safer, DJ & Zito, JM (2007) Do antidepressants reduce suicide rates? *Public Health 121*(4), 274–7.

37. Moncrieff, J (2008) The creation of the concept of the antidepressant: An historical analysis. *Social Science and Medicine, 66*, 2346–55.

Chapter 6

1. Healy, D (2008) *Mania: A short history of bipolar disorder.* Baltimore, MD: Johns Hopkins University Press.

2. Angst, J, Gamma, A, Benazzi, F, Ajdacic, V, Eich, D & Rossler, W (2003) Toward a re-definition of subthreshold bipolarity: Epidemiology and proposed criteria for bipolar II, minor bipolar disorders and hypomania. *J.Affect.Disord. 73*(1-2), 133–46.

3. Harris, M, Chandran, S, Chakraborty, N & Healy, D (2003) Mood-stabilizers: The archeology of the concept. *Bipolar.Disord. 5*(6), 446–52.

4. Barton, CD Jr, Dufer, D, Monderer, R, Cohen, MJ, Fuller, HJ, Clark, MR & DePaulo, JR Jr (1993) Mood variability in normal subjects on lithium. *Biol.Psychiatry 34*(12), 878–84.

5. Calil, HM, Zwicker, AP & Klepacz, S (1990) The effects of lithium carbonate on healthy volunteers: Mood stabilization? *Biol.Psychiatry 27*(7), 711–22.

6. Judd, LL, Hubbard, B, Janowsky, DS, Huey, LY & Takahashi, KI (1977) The effect of lithium carbonate on the cognitive functions of normal subjects. *Arch.Gen.Psychiatry 34*(3), 355–7.

7. Muller-Oerlinghausen, B, Hamann, S, Herrmann, WM & Kropf, D (1979) Effects of lithium on vigilance, psychomotoric performance and mood. *Pharmakopsychiatr.Neuropsychopharmakol. 12*(5), 388–96.

8. Prien, RF, Caffey, EM, Jr & Klett, CJ (1972) Comparison of lithium carbonate and chlorpromazine in the treatment of mania. Report of the Veterans Administration and National Institute of Mental Health Collaborative Study Group. *Arch.Gen.Psychiatry 26*(2), 146–53.

9. Braden, W, Fink, EB, Qualls, CB, Ho, CK & Samuels, WO (1982) Lithium and chlorpromazine in psychotic inpatients. *Psychiatry Res. 7*(1), 69–81.

10. See n. 8.

11. Takahashi, R, Sakuma, A, Itoh, K, Itoh, H & Kurihara, M (1975) Comparison of efficacy of lithium carbonate and chlorpromazine in mania. Report of collaborative study group on treatment of mania in Japan. *Arch.Gen.Psychiatry 32*(10), 1310–18.

12. Braden, W, Fink, EB, Qualls, CB, Ho, CK & Samuels, WO (1982), see n. 9.

13. Johnstone, EC, Crow, TJ, Frith, CD & Owens, DG (1988) The Northwick Park 'functional' psychosis study: Diagnosis and treatment response. *Lancet 2*(8603), 119–25.

14. Ibid.

15. See n. 8.

16. Chouinard, G, Young, SN & Annable, L (1983) Antimanic effect of clonazepam. *Biol.Psychiatry 18*(4), 451–66.

17. Chouinard, G (1988) The use of benzodiazepines in the treatment of manic-depressive illness. *J.Clin.Psychiatry 49* Suppl, 15–20.

18. Perlis, RH, Welge, JA, Vornik, LA, Hirschfeld, RM & Keck, PE Jr (2006) Atypical antipsychotics in the treatment of mania: A meta-analysis of randomized, placebo-controlled trials. *J.Clin.Psychiatry 67*(4), 509–16.

19. Suppes, T, Baldessarini, RJ, Faedda, GL & Tohen, M (1991) Risk of recurrence following discontinuation of lithium treatment in bipolar disorder. *Arch.Gen.Psychiatry 48*(12), 1082–8.

20. Bowden, CL, Calabrese, JR, McElroy, SL, Gyulai, L, Wassef, A, Petty, F et al (2000) A randomized, placebo-controlled 12-month trial of divalproex and lithium in treatment of outpatients with bipolar I disorder. Divalproex Maintenance Study Group. *Arch.Gen.Psychiatry 57*(5), 481–9.

21. Calabrese, JR, Bowden, CL, Sachs, G, Yatham, LN, Behnke, K, Mehtonen, OP et al (2003) A placebo-controlled 18-month trial of lamotrigine and lithium maintenance treatment in recently depressed patients with bipolar I disorder. *J.Clin.Psychiatry 64*(9), 1013–24.

22. Bowden, CL, Calabrese, JR, Sachs, G, Yatham, LN, Asghar, SA, Hompland, M et al (2003) A placebo-controlled 18-month trial of lamotrigine and lithium maintenance treatment in recently manic or hypomanic patients with bipolar I disorder. *Arch.Gen.Psychiatry 60*(4), 392–400.

23. See n. 20.

24. See n. 21.

25. See n. 22.

26. Tohen, M, Calabrese, JR, Sachs, GS, Banov, MD, Detke, HC, Risser, R et al (2006) Randomized, placebo-controlled trial of olanzapine as maintenance therapy in patients with bipolar I disorder responding to acute treatment with olanzapine. *Am.J.Psychiatry 163*(2), 247–56.

27. Bell, AJ, Cole, A, Eccleston, D & Ferrier, IN (1993) Lithium neurotoxicity at normal therapeutic levels. *Br.J.Psychiatry 162*, 689–92.

28. Gitlin, M (1999) Lithium and the kidney: An updated review. *Drug Saf. 20*(3), 231–43.

29. Kocsis, JH, Shaw, ED, Stokes, PE, Wilner, P, Elliot, AS, Sikes, C et al (1993) Neuropsychologic effects of lithium discontinuation. *J.Clin.Psychopharmacol. 13*(4), 268–75.

30. Johnston, AM & Eagles, JM (1999) Lithium-associated clinical hypothyroidism. Prevalence and risk factors. *Br.J.Psychiatry 175*, 336–9.

Chapter 7

1. Spencer, TJ, Biederman, J, Madras, BK, Faraone, SV, Dougherty, DD, Bonab, AA & Fischman, AJ (2005) In vivo neuroreceptor imaging in attention-deficit/ hyperactivity disorder: A focus on the dopamine transporter. *Biol.Psychiatry 57*(11), 1293–300.

2. Rapoport, JL, Buchsbaum, MS, Weingartner, H, Zahn, TP, Ludlow, C & Mikkelsen, EJ (1980) Dextroamphetamine. Its cognitive and behavioral effects in normal and hyperactive boys and normal men. *Arch.Gen.Psychiatry 37*(8), 933–43.

3. Breggin, PR (2001) *Talking Back to Ritalin. What doctors aren't telling you about stimulants and ADHD*. Cambridge, MA: Perseus Publishing.

4. Rie, HE, Rie, ED, Stewart, S & Ambuel, JP (1976) Effects of methylphenidate on underachieving children. *J.Consult Clin.Psychol. 44*(2), 250–60 [cited in Breggin, ibid, p 84].

5. Eichlseder, W (1985) Ten years of experience with 1,000 hyperactive children in a private practice. *Pediatrics 76*(2), 176–84.

6. Sleator, EK, Ullmann, RK & von Neumann, A (1982) How do hyperactive children feel about taking stimulants and will they tell the doctor? *Clin.Pediatr.(Phila) 21*(8), 474–9.

7. Lipkin, PH, Goldstein, IJ & Adesman, AR (1994) Tics and dyskinesias associated with stimulant treatment in attention-deficit hyperactivity disorder. *Arch.Pediatr.Adolesc.Med. 148*(8), 859–61.

8. Varley, CK, Vincent, J, Varley, P & Calderon, R (2001) Emergence of tics in children with attention deficit hyperactivity disorder treated with stimulant medications. *Compr.Psychiatry 42*(3), 228–33.

9. Askenasy, EP, Taber, KH, Yang, PB & Dafny, N (2007) Methylphenidate (Ritalin): Behavioral studies in the rat. *Int.J.Neurosci. 117*(6), 757–94.

10. Ross, DC, Fischhoff, J & Davenport, B (2002) Treatment of ADHD when tolerance to methylphenidate develops. *Psychiatr.Serv. 53*(1), 102.

11. Schachter, HM, Pham, B, King, J, Langford, S & Moher, D (2001) How efficacious and safe is short-acting methylphenidate for the treatment of attention-deficit disorder in children and adolescents? A meta-analysis. *CMAJ 165*(11), 1475–88.

12. The MTA Cooperative Group (1999) A 14-month randomized clinical trial of treatment strategies for attention-deficit/hyperactivity disorder. Multimodal Treatment Study of Children with ADHD. *Arch.Gen.Psychiatry 56*(12), 1073–86.

13. Jensen, PS, Arnold, LE, Swanson, JM, Vitiello, B, Abikoff, HB, Greenhill, LL et al (2007) Three-year follow-up of the NIMH MTA study. *J.Am.Acad.Child Adolesc.Psychiatry 46*(8), 989–1002.

14. Swanson, JM, Elliott, GR, Greenhill, LL, Wigal, T, Arnold, LE, Vitiello, B et al (2007) Effects of stimulant medication on growth rates across 3 years in the MTA follow-up. *J.Am.Acad.Child Adolesc.Psychiatry 46*(8), 1015–27.

15. Spencer, TJ, Biederman, J, Harding, M, O'Donnell, D, Faraone, SV & Wilens, TE (1996) Growth deficits in ADHD children revisited: Evidence for disorder-associated growth delays? *J.Am.Acad.Child Adolesc.Psychiatry 35*(11), 1460–9.

16. See n. 14.

17. Charach, A, Figueroa, M, Chen, S, Ickowicz, A & Schachar, R (2006) Stimulant treatment over 5 years: Effects on growth. *J.Am.Acad.Child Adolesc.Psychiatry 45*(4), 415–21.

18. Royal College of Psychiatrists (2004) *Stimulant Medication for ADHD and Hyperkinetic Disorder.* London: Royal College of Psychiatrists.

19. See n. 3.

20. Pizzi, WJ, Rode, EC & Barnhart, JE (1986) Methylphenidate and growth: Demonstration of a growth impairment and a growth-rebound phenomenon. *Dev.Pharmacol.Ther. 9*(5), 361–8.

21. Klein, RG & Mannuzza, S (1988) Hyperactive boys almost grown up. III. Methylphenidate effects on ultimate height. *Arch.Gen.Psychiatry 45*(12), 1131–4.

22. Nissen, SE (2006) ADHD drugs and cardiovascular risk. *N.Engl.J.Med. 354*(14), 1445–8.

23. Nissen, SE (2006) Letter to the Editor. *New England Journal of Medicine 354*, 2296.

24. Elkins, IJ, McGue, M & Iacono, WG (2007) Prospective effects of attention-deficit/hyperactivity disorder, conduct disorder, and sex on adolescent substance use and abuse. *Arch.Gen.Psychiatry 64*(10), 1145–52.

25. Wilens, TE, Faraone, SV, Biederman, J & Gunawardene, S (2003) Does stimulant therapy of attention-deficit/hyperactivity disorder beget later substance abuse? A meta-analytic review of the literature. *Pediatrics 111*(1), 179–85.

26. Biederman, J, Wilens, T, Mick, E, Spencer, T & Faraone, SV (1999) Pharmacotherapy of attention-deficit/hyperactivity disorder reduces risk for substance use disorder. *Pediatrics 104*(2), e20.

27. Lambert, N (2007) The contribution of childhood ADHD, conduct problems, and stimulant treatment to adolescent and adult tobacco and psychoactive substance abuse. *Ethical Human Psychology and Psychiatry 7*(3), 197–221.

28. Molina, BS, Flory, K, Hinshaw, SP, Greiner, AR, Arnold, LE, Swanson, JM et al (2007) Delinquent behavior and emerging substance use in the MTA at 36 months: Prevalence, course, and treatment effects. *J.Am.Acad.Child Adolesc.Psychiatry 46*(8), 1028–40.

29. A Z-test of the difference between two proportions yields a Z value of 1.83, and a two-tailed p value of 0.07, just above the conventional 0.05 level of statistical significance.

30. Whalen, CK & Henker, B (1976) Psychostimulants and children: A review and analysis. *Psychol.Bull. 83*(6), 1113–30.

31. Thorley, G (1988) Adolescent outcome for hyperactive children. *Arch.Dis.Child 63*(10), 1181–3.

32. Valentine, M (1988) *How to Deal with Difficult Discipline Problems: A family systems approach.* Dubuque, IA: Kendall Hunt publishing company.

Chapter 8

1. Nutt, DJ & Malizia, AL (2001) New insights into the role of the GABA(A)-benzodiazepine receptor in psychiatric disorder. *Br.J.Psychiatry 179*, 390–6.

2. Ashton, H (1987) Benzodiazepine withdrawal: Outcome in 50 patients. *Br.J.Addict. 82*(6), 665–71.

3. Golombok, S, Moodley, P & Lader, M (1988) Cognitive impairment in long-term benzodiazepine users. *Psychol.Med. 18*(2), 365–74.

4. Lader, MH, Ron, M & Petursson, H (1984) Computed axial brain tomography in long-term benzodiazepine users. *Psychol.Med. 14*(1), 203–6.

5. Schmauss, C & Krieg, JC (1987) Enlargement of cerebrospinal fluid spaces in long-term benzodiazepine abusers. *Psychol.Med. 17*(4), 869–73.

6. Busto, UE, Bremner, KE, Knight, K, terBrugge, K & Sellers, EM (2000) Long-term benzodiazepine therapy does not result in brain abnormalities. *J.Clin.Psychopharmacol. 20*(1), 2–6.

7. Perera, KM, Powell, T & Jenner, FA (1987) Computerized axial tomographic studies following long-term use of benzodiazepines. *Psychol.Med. 17*(3), 775–7.

8. Taylor, D, Paton, C & Kerwin, R (2005) *The Maudsley 2005–2006 Prescribing Guidelines.* London: Taylor & Francis.

9. Carpenter, WT Jr, Buchanan, RW, Kirkpatrick, B & Breier, AF (1999) Diazepam treatment of early signs of exacerbation in schizophrenia. *Am.J.Psychiatry 156*(2), 299–303.

Chapter 9

1. Moncrieff, J (2008) *The Myth of the Chemical Cure: A critique of psychiatric drug treatment.* Basingstoke: Palgrave Macmillan.

2. Pfizer (2006) Accessed February 6, 2006 at www.geodon.com/s_WhatCauses.asp

3. Eli Lilly (2006) Accessed 10 February 2006 at www.prozac.com/how_prozac/how_it_works.jsp?reqNavId=2.2

4. Eli Lilly (2009) How Zyprexa (olanzapine) works. Accessed 26 February 2009 at http://www.zyprexa.com/sch/learnaboutzyprexa/howzyprexaworks.jsp

Chapter 10

1. Moncrieff, J (2006) Does antipsychotic withdrawal provoke psychosis? Review of the literature on rapid onset psychosis (supersensitivity psychosis) and withdrawal-related relapse. *Acta Psychiatr.Scand. 114*(1), 3–13.

2. Suppes, T, Baldessarini, RJ, Faedda, GL & Tohen, M (1991) Risk of recurrence following discontinuation of lithium treatment in bipolar disorder. *Arch.Gen.Psychiatry 48*(12), 1082–8.

3. Viguera, AC, Baldessarini, RJ, Hegarty, JD, van Kammen, DP & Tohen, M (1997) Clinical risk following abrupt and gradual withdrawal of maintenance neuroleptic treatment. *Arch.Gen.Psychiatry 54*(1), 49–55.

Chapter 11

1. Page 76 in Breggin, PR (1997) *Brain Disabling Treatments in Psychiatry: Drugs, electroshock and the role of the FDA.* New York: Springer Publishing Company.

Appendix
Sources of information about stopping and reducing psychiatric drugs

Coming Off Psychiatric Medication website. www.comingoff.com

Harm Reduction Guide to Coming off Psychiatric Drugs. Published by Icarus Project and Freedom Center, USA, 2007. Available for download from www.theicarusproject.net/alternativetreatments/harm-reduction-guide-to-coming-off-psychiatric-drugs

Making sense of coming off psychiatric drugs. Published by Mind, London, UK, 2005. Available at http://www.mind.org.uk/Information/Booklets/Making+sense/Making+sense+of+coming+off+psychiatric+drugs.htm

Your Drug May Be Your Problem: How and why to stop taking psychiatric medication (1999) P Breggin & D Cohen. Published by Perseus Books, Cambridge, MA, USA.

Subject Index

Index

Index

Name Index

Psychiatric drugs

Psychiatric drugs